The Truly Dynamic Therapist

Jacquelyne Morison

authorHOUSE®

AuthorHouse™ UK Ltd.
500 Avebury Boulevard
Central Milton Keynes, MK9 2BE
www.authorhouse.co.uk
Phone: 08001974150

First published by AuthorHouse 12/17/2008

ISBN: 978-1-4343-2700-0 (sc)

Library of Congress Control Number: 2007908355

Printed in the United States of America
Bloomington, Indiana

This book is printed on acid-free paper.

DEDICATION

To Marianne Callaghan and Susanne Elbrond and to all my enthusiastic, open-hearted, awe-inspiring and wonderful contributors.

ACKNOWLEDGEMENTS

I would like to warmly thank those practitioners who have so willingly and touchingly helped me to compile case-study examples and/or allowed me to gain insight into certain areas of the alternative therapy field. The main contributors to and/or sources of inspiration for this book cover a vast range of therapeutic disciplines and those of special note are listed below.

Barbara Akers, *Counselor*; **Claire Auger**, *Colonic Hydrotherapist, Massage Therapist, Reflexologist*; **Natalie Bachet**, *Acupuncturist*; **Judie Barnes**, *Reflexologist*; **Linda Barr**, *Nutritionist*; **John Bayford**, *Acupuncturist, Nutritionist, Quantum Shen Therapist, Shiatsu Practitioner*; **Susan Berry**, *Homeopath*; **John Boulderstone**, *Craniosacral Therapist, Homeopath, Life Force Healer, Yoga Teacher*; **Liolah Boysen**, *Art Therapist, Counselor*; **Brian Browne**, *Psychotherapist*; **Anne Bryson**, *Hypnotherapist*; **Catherine Burton**, *Indian Head Massage Therapist, Massage Therapist, Reflexologist*; **Marianne Callaghan**, *Kinesiologist, Nutritionist*; **Charlotte Chalkley**, *Hypnotherapist*; **Howard Charing**, *Shamanic Healer*; **Paul Cheneour**, *Meditation Facilitator*; **Gail Clarke**, *Alexander Technique Teacher*; **Allan Clifford**, *Bowen Technique Practitioner*; **Andrew Cook**, *Craniosacral Therapist, Osteopath*; **Julian Cowan Hill**, *Craniosacral Therapist*; **Jo Crowe**, *Shamanic Healer*; **Binnie Dansby**, *Rebirthing Therapist*; **Graham Davies**, *Indian Head Massage Therapist, Life Coach, Meditation Facilitator, Spiritual Healer*; **Chris D-Cruz**, *Nutritionist, Rebirthing Therapist*; **Max Delli Guanti**, *Counselor, Hypnotherapist*; **Carol Dowle**, *Chiropractor*; **Gail Duff**, *Rebirthing Therapist, Reiki Healer*; **Angie Dyson**, *Colonic Hydrotherapist*; **Cris Edwards**, *Hypnotherapist*; **Susanne Elbrond**, *Craniosacral Therapist*; **Andrew Elliott**, *Acupuncturist*; **Susan Fairley**, *Aura Soma Therapist, Craniosacral Therapist, Osteopath*; **Marian Farrell**, *Hypnotherapist, Reiki Healer, Spiritual Psychotherapist*; **Bill Ferguson**, *Acupuncturist, Osteopath*; **Mary Ann Findlay**, *Homeopath*; **Marianne Friend**, *Massage Therapist, Rebirthing Therapist, Spiritual Healer*; **Stuart Frost**, *Counselor, Hypnotherapist, Reiki Healer*; **Steve Frost**, *Shamanic Healer*; **John Gavin**, *Acupuncturist, Chinese Herbalist, Naturopath, Reflexologist*; **Catherine Glanfield**, *Homeopath*; **Wendy Glassock**, *Massage Therapist, Reflexologist*; **Anthony Gorman**, *Spiritual Healer*;

Lynn Gosney, *Shamanic Healer*; **Tom Greenfield**, *Blood Group Consultant, Craniosacral Therapist, Naturopath, Osteopath*; **Jeannie Harkett**, *Immuno-Lymphatic Therapist*; **Nicola Harvey**, *Colonic Hydrotherapist*; **Eliana Harvey**, *Shamanic Healer*; **Sarah Hayward**, *Chiropractor*; **Rachel Henderson**, *Emotional Freedom Technique Therapist, Hypnotherapist, Reiki Healer*; **Christina Horton**, *Colonic Hydrotherapist*; **Suzette Hughes**, *Homeopath, Psychotherapist*; **Susan Hughes**, *Psychotherapist, Reiki Healer*; **Joe Keaney**, *Hypnotherapist*; **Michael Kern**, *Craniosacral Therapist, Naturopath, Osteopath*; **Judith King**, *Counselor, Massage Therapist, Thermo-Auricular Therapist*; **Kay Lakka**, *Psychotherapist*; **Judy Lamb**, *Emotional Freedom Technique Therapist, Indian Head Massage Therapist, Metaphysical Counselor, Reflexologist*; **Brian Lamb**, *Counselor, Naturopath*; **Olga Lawrence Jones**, *Counselor, Homeopath*; **Alison Lees**, *Homeopath, Shamanic Healer*; **Li Li**, *Acupuncturist, Chinese Herbalist, Reflexologist*; **Jun Li**, *Acupuncturist, Chinese Herbalist, Reflexologist*; **Brenda Loach**, *Bowen Technique Practitioner*; **Eileen Ludlow**, *Hypnotherapist, Integrated Energies Therapist, Reflexologist, Reiki Healer*; **Kathie Mabberley**, *Bowen Technique Practitioner, Craniosacral Therapist*; **Salvina Macari**, *Reflexologist*; **Tsenka Mack**, *Osteopath*; **Manisha Makwana-Soneji**, *Craniosacral Therapist, Hypnotherapist, Massage Therapist, Nutritionist*; **Lorna Marchant**, *Kinesiologist, Nutritionist*; **Sue Marshall**, *Pilates Teacher, Yoga Teacher*; **Lynn Marsh-Jones**, *Hypnotherapist*; **Bridget McCabe**, *Homeopath, Vibrational Medicine Practitioner*; **Neil McCarthy**, *Shiatsu Practitioner*; **Madelene McConomy**, *Iridologist*; **Donna Milton**, *Hypnotherapist*; **Ian Molloy**, *Emotional Freedom Technique Therapist, Hypnotherapist*; **Alysson Moore**, *Craniosacral Therapist, Massage Therapist*; **Milena Moore**, *Medical Herbalist*; **Farid Moshtael**, *Chiropractor*; **Pamela Mousley**, *Homeopath*; **Joke Murray**, *Assemblage Point Therapist, Energy Medicine Therapist, Shiatsu Practitioner, Yoga Teacher*; **Lesley Murray**, *Homeopath*; **Jacqui Murray**, *Hypnotherapist*; **Ara Alexis Nafari**, *Chiropractor*; **Philippa Nice**, *Acupuncturist*; **Heather Nicholson**, *Iridologist, Nutritionist*; **Peter O'Loughlin**, *Counselor, Psychotherapist*; **Gail Palmer**, *Craniosacral Therapist, Medical Herbalist*; **Lorraine Parker**, *Counselor, Hypnotherapist*; **Alison Parrington**, *Counselor, Homeopath*; **Elise Paterson**, *Massage Therapist, Reflexologist*; **Jill Payne**, *Alexander Technique*

Teacher; **Vera Peiffer**, *Kinesiologist, Psychotherapist*; **Philip Pelham**, *Medical Herbalist*; **Andri Pelle**, *Hypnotherapist*; **Georges Philips**, *Hypnotherapist, Life Coach*; **Lyn Philips**, *Hypnotherapist, Psychic Healer, Spiritual Psychotherapist*; **Christopher Pieri**, *Bates Vision Teacher, Bowen Technique Practitioner, Naturopath*; **Sandra Pledger**, *Indian Head Massage Therapist, Reiki Healer, Thermo-Auricular Therapist*; **Mike Rawlinson**, *Alexander Technique Teacher*; **Charles Read**, *Osteopath*; **Susan Reeves**, *Emotional Freedom Technique Therapist, Reflexologist, Thermo-Auricular Therapist*; **Mary Robertson**, *Counselor, Psychotherapist*; **Philip Roe**, *Osteopath*; **Leslie Ross**, *Acupuncturist*; **Leo Rutherford**, *Shamanic Healer*; **Terence Shadwell**, *Psychotherapist*; **Fiona Shields**, *Psychotherapist, Reflexologist, Reiki Healer, Vibrational Medicine Practitioner*; **Fiona Silk**, *Medical Herbalist*; **Franklyn Sills**, *Craniosacral Therapist, Osteopath, Polarity Therapist*; **Maggie Smith**, *Counselor*; **Keith Smith**, *Homeopath, Life Coach*; **Maree Smith**, *Massage Therapist, Nutritionist, Reflexologist, Thermo-Auricular Therapist*; **Sally Stonier**, *Color Healer, Dance Therapist, Rebirthing Therapist, Reiki Healer*; **Deborah Summers**, *Infant Massage Therapist, Massage Therapist*; **Jane Taylor**, *Craniosacral Therapist, Spiritual Healer*; **Julie Thatcher**, *Indian Head Massage Therapist*; **Anne Todd**, *Emotional Freedom Technique Therapist*; **Cathy Tredgett**, *Astrologer*; **Caroline Turk**, *Osteopath*; **Linda Turner**, *Spiritual Response Therapist*; **Sara Turner**, *Vibrational Medicine Practitioner*; **Rebecca Vann**, *Indian Head Massage Therapist, Pilates Teacher, Reiki Healer, Yoga Teacher*; **Lucy Vertue**, *Craniosacral Therapist, Medical Herbalist*; **Elaine Walker**, *Homeopath*; **Tania Waller**, *Crystal Healer, Metamorphic Technique Practitioner, Reflexologist, Reiki Healer*; **Linda Wilson**, *Acupuncturist, Massage Therapist*; **Richard West**, *Environmental Healer, Reiki Healer, Spiritual Healer*; **Vincent Winter**, *Geopathic Stress Consultant, Space Clearing Consultant*; **Michelle Wolfe-Emery**, *Spiritual Psychotherapist*.

I am indebted to all my students at the **International College of Eclectic Therapies** in London who have made a generous and significant contribution to this work. I am, also, grateful to all those students and course delegates whom I have met through my work at the **Institute of Clinical Hypnotherapy and Psychotherapy** in the Republic of Ireland and, especially, to those who have so willingly and patiently helped me with writing this book. All practitioners who have received supervision from me have, of course, provided a rich source of inspiration for this book and I, hereby, express my eternal gratitude.

I would wish to acknowledge the help that I have received from the practitioners and staff at the **Counseling Service at the University of Kent at Canterbury, Forstal Holistic Health, Karmers Centre, Number 11 Complementary Therapy Centre** and **Spring Gardens Clinic**.

I would finally wish to mention the support and cooperation that I have received from a number of professional bodies, as given below, in connection with my research for this book.

The Association of Analytical and Cognitive Therapists, the Association of Reflexologists, the Association of Systematic Kinesiology, the Bowen Association UK, the Bowen Therapists' European Register, the British Acupuncture Council, the British Association for Nutritional Therapy, the British Chiropractic Association, the British Flower and Vibrational Essences Association, the British Holistic Medical Association, the British Medical Acupuncture Society, the British Rebirth Society, the Complementary Medical Association, the Craniosacral Therapy Association of the UK, the General Chiropractic Council, the General Hypnotherapy Register, the General Osteopathic Council, the Guild of Complementary Therapists, the Guild of Naturopathic Iridologists International, Health Kinesiology UK, the Homeopathic Medical Association, the Hypnotherapy Society, the Institute of Optimum Nutrition, the International Federation of Professional Aromatherapists, the International Register of Consultant Medical Herbalists and Homoeopaths, the International Reiki Federation, the Kinesiology Federation, Manual Lymphatic Drainage UK, the McTimoney Chiropractic Association, the National Council for Hypnotherapy, the National Institute of Ayurvedic Medicine, the National Institute of Medical Herbalists, the Register of Chinese Herbal Medicine, the Shiatsu Society, the Society of Celtic Shamans, the Society of Homeopaths, the Society of Teachers of the Alexander Technique and the United Chiropractic Association.

JAM

CONTENTS

FOREWORD

With her latest book, *The Truly Dynamic Therapist*, Jacquelyne Morison presents a thought-provoking analysis of modern alternative therapy in all its facets. The book not only looks at a plethora of alternative therapies but also explores every angle of practitioner development.

Jacquelyne takes a holistic approach to treatment, covering not only psychological aspects of therapy but also physical and spiritual ones that can help unravel a client's physical and emotional suffering by rooting out the underlying causes. The book challenges the established therapist to scrutinize their attitude towards themselves and their clients. Practitioners are encouraged to adopt a more wide-ranging view of alternative therapy treatments, one that encompasses more than just one discipline. As Jacquelyne points out, human beings are complex and multifaceted, and, therefore, their healing has to be able to address the many layers of the problem a client is seeking help with.

An accomplished alternative practitioner herself, Jacquelyne has over the years acquired an impressive array of skills as a hypnotherapist, craniosacral, nutritional therapist and energetic healer. Having herself undergone an even vaster range of alternative therapies on her path of recovery from illness and depression has enabled her to produce a truly amazing piece of work. *The Truly Dynamic Therapist* is based on intimate knowledge of alternative therapies and of questions a therapist will have to ask themselves if they want to progress in their personal and professional development.

In contrast to the many quick-fix manuals that are churned out every year by publishers, Jacquelyne goes deeper, probes more uncomfortably and asks more searching questions. She encourages practitioners to become the best therapists they can possibly be by getting to the root of their clients' (and, also, their own) limitations and stumbling blocks.

Packed with real-life examples and case histories, *The Truly Dynamic Therapist* does not only support practitioners in their quest for more effective ways to help others, it also looks at practical issues such as practice set-up, promotional material and advertising.

I have no doubt that this book will become an invaluable handbook for both those planning on starting a career as an alternative practitioner and for those already in practice. This is a book full of wisdom and compassion that needs to be read over and over again. *The Truly Dynamic Therapist* may well be the greatest asset in your personal and professional development that you have ever invested in!

Vera Peiffer

WHAT IS THIS BOOK ALL ABOUT?

What will be in this book for you?

Because alternative and complementary medicine has not been given its full credit, sadly the role of the alternative practitioner has not been recognized, has not been considered to be particularly important and has, therefore, not been written about much. The premise of *The Truly Dynamic Therapist* will be to explore, in depth, the entire spectrum of the healing journey that you will take as a therapeutic practitioner from inception to retirement. This book will take you on a voyage of self-questioning and thought-provoking analysis of yourself, your life, your work and your clientele in search of the solution that will be exactly right for you and for you alone. *The Truly Dynamic Therapist* will, consequently, be your passport to being and evolving as an alternative practitioner.

Part 1 – YOU AND ALTERNATIVE THERAPY will consider the role and nature of alternative therapy and complementary medicine so that you can neatly dovetail yourself into the holistic matrix with insight. Here you can, also, gain your inspiration from the philosophies of others. This part of the book will explain the premise that underpins alternative therapeutic practice and its importance as the ultimate healing profession.

Part 2 – YOU AND YOUR CLIENT will examine, in detail, the vital ingredients of alternative therapy – the relationship that you will form with yourself as an individual and the way in which you will interact with your client. This section of the book will help you to explore the principal substance of your evolutionary journey. Here you can put yourself under the microscope in order to discover and enhance your strengths and to overcome any weakness all of which will be a vital part of your professional development.

Part 3 – YOU AND YOUR BUSINESS will deal with the nitty-gritty of launching your therapeutic practice and, then, keeping your business afloat from a practical viewpoint. This part of the book will serve to stimulate your creativity with regard to professional self-promotion and business management.

What might be the supreme tragedy of our age?

There may be many replies to this question but, for me, there can only be one ultimate answer. The supreme tragedy of the last millennium, and, possibly, this one, might be the fact that only a minute minority of people actually recognize that the sole key to the optimal health of the human system must be via alternative therapy. That is to say, for optimal health, your client's system will usually need to undergo a total detoxification procedure in order to heal her body-tissue, her biochemical distress, her physical malfunction and her emotional trauma as well as allowing her to climb towards spiritual self-awareness. This cleansing process may, also, require your client to return to the source of her disorder and, perhaps, even to the moment of conception, if necessary, in order to trace her malaise back through any historical inheritances from previous generations. But this will be where you, as an alternative practitioner, will come into the equation with full force.

Only by adhering to and by worshipping the natural self-healing process, can the inhabitants of planet earth ever hope to achieve healthy functioning, recover from illness, prevent both everyday malaise and killer diseases, enjoy maximal longevity, attain emotional stability, reach relationship harmony and bring about freedom from all those ills that collectively beset the nations of the world. Alternative therapy, as a universal curative and preventive measure, will ensure that our worldwide spiraling ill-health, our universal dissatisfaction, our multi-national unrest and our epidemic proportions of misconceptions about health-care are not handed down and perpetuated in future generations. Although clinical evidence in alternative practice may have proven its efficacy, even beyond the disbelief of scientific skepticism, the stigma attached to alternative therapy, regrettably, still persists today in a society encrusted with ignorance.

Why would I get on my soap-box?

Let me occupy your time for a moment by quoting from my own personal narrative. Alternative therapy and complementary medicine have, in short, saved my life. I am sure that my case cannot be unique or that different from those of other sufferers and, perhaps, you may be one or have been one.

I suffered from a lifelong history of suicidal depression that reached its peak during my so-called mid-life crisis when I became crippled with what was casually and summarily termed as an arthritic condition. I was unable to walk any distance without being in excruciating agony both at the time and for days afterwards. It, then, took me about ten years or so of hard labor in order to cut through the barbed wire towards freedom. I had to endure the agony of unwinding my biochemical, my physiological and my psychological history and this work has enabled me to arrive at a semblance of order.

My life had, back in the bad old days, come to a complete standstill in every way. Initially I drew in my horns in order to relieve the pain and the torment. Once I had been forced to take the decision to unwind the tangle, I, then, set about seeking a mixture of alternative and orthodox assistance. Without exception, all the orthodox medicine, together with the manipulative and surgical intervention that I endured, only made matters worse and stacked up for me even more devastating disaster. When I turned to alternative practice, I was, then, well on my way to unraveling the mess. Even so, I still had to be selective in finding those therapeutic practitioners who not only suited my temperament and my personality but also who possessed the depth of knowledge, the personal experience, the guts and the sheer bloody-minded determination to ignore my symptoms and go all out for the

3

originating cause. In a nutshell, the combined underlying causes were devastating. Repressed childhood trauma of neglect, violence and abuse accounted for my emotional ill-health and, in addition, medical and surgical intervention, coupled with systemic pollution, had reduced me to a helpless cripple.

I have spent, to date, more than a decade ploughing through the agonizing ordeal of restoring my emotional health and physical wellbeing, not to mention a very well-spent financial fortune into the bargain. I have, also, had to screw my courage to the sticking post with a crazy mixture of teeth-gritting resolve and blind faith in order to pull myself though with the zealous tenacity of a turbo-charged maniac, despite almost impossible odds. My journey along the alternative path has taken me principally via analytical hypnotherapy, craniosacral therapy, nutritional medicine, kinesiology, homeopathy and spiritual healing. This fundamental core of therapies has been augmented by a hefty sprinkling of other practices, such as acupuncture, the Alexander technique, assemblage point therapy, bioresonance, Bates vision therapy, Bowen technique, buteyko, chiropractic, colonic hydrotherapy, color healing, counseling, crystal healing, emotional freedom technique therapy, flower essences, herbal medicine, Indian head massage, iridology, massage therapy, meditation, naturopathy, osteopathy, the Pilates method, polarity therapy, psychotherapy, rebirthing, reflexology, reiki healing, shamanic healing, shiatsu massage, sound healing, Thai massage, thought field therapy and yoga, to name but a few. This path has been an arduous uphill struggle for me, and it is not over yet, but my experience has made me a lifelong devotee and exponent of the natural root to restoring optimal health.

Inevitably, my dedication to the process has seen me become qualified as a hypnotherapist, a craniosacral therapist, a nutritional therapist and an energetic healer and, like most alternative practitioners, I have signed the pledge of a lifetime's commitment to being and living the life of a healer. My work as a practitioner, a supervisor, a teacher and an author has lead to the creation of this book. I, therefore, sincerely hope that you will enjoy and benefit from the fruits of my labors, picked up along my own personal healing path.

PART 1
YOU AND ALTERNATIVE THERAPY

1 WHAT WOULD CONSTITUTE ILL-HEALTH?

How would the world explain the phenomenon of ill-health?

How misguided might the man in the street be about ill-health? When we encounter something that we cannot immediately explain in a logical way, our mind will ingeniously invent a suitable alternative that satisfies the curiosity. The mysterious phenomenon and curse of ill-health will, therefore, be a prime target for worldwide irrational speculation.

What will the unenlightened public believe?
The vast majority of people probably believe that some malicious and scheming god sits in a diamond-encrusted, ivory tower and decides our fate as an amusing pastime. This omnipotent being will randomly scatter his lethal magic darts from above the stratosphere and they will, then, land on any poor, unsuspecting victim at the chance spin of an invisible roulette wheel. Hence disease, illness, disorder, degeneration, emotional disharmony and general somatic malfunction are born along with old age, senility and irrational behavioral tendencies. This may be the way in which we usually can explain the baffling occurrence and inevitable presence of disease in our society. Friends may offer sympathy and, sometimes, well-meaning, albeit unhelpful, advice to the afflicted. The sufferer will, then, become resigned to an inevitable fate with nothing to do about it but to complain.

This blinkered view of ill-health, of course, is nonsensical, despite the fact that this may be precisely what most people sincerely believe. There could really be no such thing as disease in the sense that it might be perceived by the man in the street. Your client's arthritis, her cancer, her heart disease or her late-onset diabetes, for example, are all conditions that will develop when her immune system has been rendered totally unable to deal with an overload of toxicity in her body and this state has, consequently, affected her vital organs and her metabolic performance. Your client's alcoholism, her anxiety, her depression or her lack of confidence, similarly, are not disorders that will afflict the unwary but will be conditions that can arise due to her past stressful or traumatic experience when her system's emotional responses and her biochemistry have been overwhelmed. Your client's allergies, her asthma, her excessive perspiration, her irritable bowel syndrome or her skin conditions, moreover, can be induced by her stress, although relieved or stilled by addressing her emotional issues, her biochemical imbalances and her energetic disturbances. The resolution of all these ills, of course, will add up to the need to address the root cause of your client's disorder rather than merely suppressing her symptoms and so treating her body as if it were a malfunctioning mechanical contraption. The tragedy and scandal of the age, then, might be that we wonder why ill-health strikes. An even greater misfortune may be that very few people truly understand the fundamental concept of why so-called disease disorders manifest in the first place.

Let's look at it another way – Life without soap

Many people believe that washing without soap will be next door to being immoral. The masses fervently believe that for so-called hygienic reasons, it will be vital to use daily the amount of soap that would normally suffice for a whole week. Are we such a world of filthy reprobates that we need to embalm ourselves in a daily soap-mountain? Advertisements for soap often show a person using enough soap to wash an entire army of people. Such advertisements may depict soap voluminously cascading out of the shower, coating the bathroom floor and voluptuously engorging the bather in a layer of foam thicker than a fur-coat suitable for arctic temperatures.

ᅟ

Soap is, however, a heavy-duty commodity. The average bar of soap may contain harmful chemicals, bleaching agents, foaming agents, colorants and perfumes that might conceivably be appropriate for a coal-miner but are actually harmful to the average body. Soap with such ingredients will clog the skin's pores and will even prevent the skin, as a major detoxifying organ, from fulfilling its natural cleansing function. If you are servicing the car or are clearing out the coal-shed, then, there may be an argument for using a little soap the next time you have a shower. But beware of employing the proverbial sledgehammer to crack the nut on a daily basis.

We do not need soap in order to live. Soap can do more harm than good. A daily bath or a shower in warm water will do the intended job even more efficiently than any soap as a heavy-weight product. The skin's own ecological system will remove any perspiration and grime very efficiently with the help of only a little water. Why kill those good guys on the skin that naturally cleanse the body? Skin irritations may abound because of the regular application of harmful agents directly on to the skin's surface. For the health-conscious person, soap might be unthinkable but many would regard life without soap as a fate worse than death itself. To those who know the secret of the non-soap regime, the logic will be obvious and self-evident. But how would you try explaining these enlightening facts to the great unwashed?

Let's take an example – Silvia's story

Silvia's principal worry was a feeling of welling anger that frequently erupted towards her family. Silvia was, also, a long-term sufferer from insomnia that merely added to her daytime anxieties. Silvia initially sought massage therapy and herbal remedies as a means of dealing with her anger because she felt that she needed to calm herself down.

After some time and success with alternative medicine, Silvia decided to undertake a course of psychotherapy. This investigation brought to light Silvia's fundamental issues with regard to being separated from her family in childhood. Silvia spent many years at boarding school in one country while her parents resided in another. The result was that Silvia could not form a bond with her parents who, in any case, were dictatorial, bigoted and controlling towards her and her siblings. This stage of Silvia's healing journey was pivotal and allowed her to release her pent-up anger and to realize its true source.

Silvia, then, elected to look into acupuncture and craniosacral therapy as a means of dealing with her sleeping disorder and, by this means, she *found relief from her underlying anxieties that had prevented her from sleeping and getting regular rest. Finally, Silvia undertook a program of nutritional cleansing in order to deal with an eating disorder and a weight problem that she had, hitherto, been ignoring and denying.*

How would you take an overview of your client's health?

Will you capture the whole picture of your client? In treating your client within your own therapeutic discipline, you will need to realize that a multiplicity of factors can enter the equation all of which will contribute to her ill-health. Having an appreciation of those related factors concerned with your client's condition will enable you to take the detached overview rather than the much-to-be-avoided narrowly-focused and closed-minded approach.

What will you behold when you meet your client?

The holographic being, known as your client, can never really be fully understood and, so, the very best you can hope for will be to gain just a glimpse into this unfathomable entity.

You may need to truly appreciate that your client will consist of a physical body comprising cells, tissue, organs and integrated systems, a mind with its emotions, cognition and mentality, an extraordinarily complex biochemical factory and a number of subtle energetic fields. All these facets of your client will record her past experiences and her genetic history as well as holding her current life-story. Your client as a live, human creature, moreover, will continually undergo a process of ingesting and assimilating nutrients, the waste-products of which must be expelled in order to generate energy and to ensure her continued existence as well as permitting cellular reproduction. Your client will, of course, express emotions, feel compelled to adopt certain behavioral patterns and be susceptible to sensation as well as being able to reason, reflect, acquire and apply knowledge.

An overview of your client's health, with the above factors in mind, will tell you, therefore, whether she will be generating

health or degenerating due either to factors beyond her control
or to self-inflicted punishment. Your client may be going against
the grain because she will be psychologically motivated to self-
destruct or she may simply be ill-informed. Your job will be to
decipher her motivations, to discover the route cause of her dilemma and, then, to steer her gently towards getting on the right
track.

Ask yourself . . .

*Can you stand back and take an overview of your client's symptoms
and her overall state of health? Can you fully appreciate that your client
will be a multi-faceted being? Will you acknowledge that aspects of your
client's being are beyond her understanding? Could your client begin
to realize that her disorder will be a complex combination of factors?
Could your client appreciate that the label that her condition has been
given may not be appropriate or even necessary? Does your client have
any inkling about why her condition has arisen? Will your client understand that her physical malaise may be aggravated by a poor diet or a
hectic lifestyle? Does your client realize that emotional factors can play
a significant role in the development of her disease and can impede her
recovery process? Could your client appreciate that her state of mind will
adversely affect her health and her general outlook? Could your client
consider that her unhappy social relationships have led her to a self-punishing lifestyle regime? Does your client rely on believing that all her
ill-health has been inherited? Can your client conceive that there will
not be a trite explanation for her condition that she could merely have
obtained off-pat from a popular magazine? Does your client realize that
her susceptibility to infectious disease may be the result of an overload of
environmental, physiological and psychological toxicity? In what ways
might your client be attempting to kill herself or to foreshorten her life?
To which harmful and irritating agents has your client been continually
exposed? Can your client appreciate that her symptoms are not necessarily indicative of the originating cause of her disease? Can you appreciate
that your client may need to consult a practitioner in a related area, or in
an entirely different field, if she is to secure effective progress?*

Let's take an example – Octavia's story

Octavia works in the field of nutrition and kinesiology and part of her work involves being accurately able to diagnose her client's needs. On many occasions, therefore, Octavia would arrive at the conclusion that a given client would need to see someone else and that, therefore, she should be referred to another practitioner. Often her client would be advised to see a psychotherapeutic practitioner or a physical therapist, despite the fact that these were disciplines utterly outside Octavia's field of operation.

The problem with this course of action frequently resulted in Octavia's client being reluctant to take her advice. Perhaps Octavia's client would not be willing to see a given therapist in a completely different discipline or would not take the initiative to find a suitable practitioner. On occasion, the practitioner to whom Octavia had referred her client was, in fact, not willing to or unable to provide the necessary treatment. Difficulties began to mount, therefore, because some of Octavia's clients were not making the much-hoped-for progress.

Octavia, then, found a solution to her dilemma by explaining carefully to all her new clients that referral to another practitioner might need to be an integral part of her treatment. Octavia emphasized that progress could only be made if her client were to comply with her recommendation when necessary. Furthermore, Octavia decided to distance herself from those clients who did not pursue her recommendation to see a practitioner in another field. Octavia, thus, refused to see any client who was not being cooperative in taking the initiative to bring about her own self-healing via the recommended route. By this means, Octavia, then, gained maximum job-satisfaction because she was, now, cherry-picking her clients.

What would be the complex matrix of your client's ill-health?

How will the spider's web of your client's ill-health be woven? Your client's ill-health might be a condition that will have developed because her system has been exposed to toxicity and trauma that can, as a knock-on effect, result in a biochemical, physiological and/or psychological imbalance or deficiency. This state will, then, inevitably have an adverse effect on your client's whole functioning. The originating cause of your client's malaise may stem from a number of internal and external sources that may be many and varied and that will frequently combine to cause her ill-health. Your client's health problems, therefore, may stem from a whole collection of sources concerned with her genetic inheritance, her physiological trauma, her psychologically-damaging experience, her environmental pollution, her biochemical toxicity, her metabolic inefficiency and her weakened immunity, coupled with her exposure to any pathogenic disease (see Figure 1.1 – *Where might your client's ill-health originate?*).

Perhaps you can pause for a moment in order to consider your client's overall health picture by not confining your thoughts to your immediate interest in terms of the specific alternative therapy that you practice. Once you have gained a clear understanding of your client's overall health picture, this knowledge may prevent you from blaming yourself when you feel you have failed to conjure up a miracle-cure.

What will be your client's genetic profile?

Every human creature on the planet will possess some form of genetic defect because man has been on the earth for some time now. Your client will arrive in your consulting room, therefore, with a number of known and/or unknown inherited factors all of which she may be required to address.

Your client's generic inheritance, of course, will impact largely on the way in which you can help her to tackle her health disorders. Detective work on your part will endeavor to establish whether any genetic disorders are a genuine threat to your client's wellbeing and, thus, will need to be supported in a conducive environment rather than being totally cured. Your client could feel that her inheritance will be a cross that she must bear but, perhaps, in truth, her condition could easily be managed to a tolerable level.

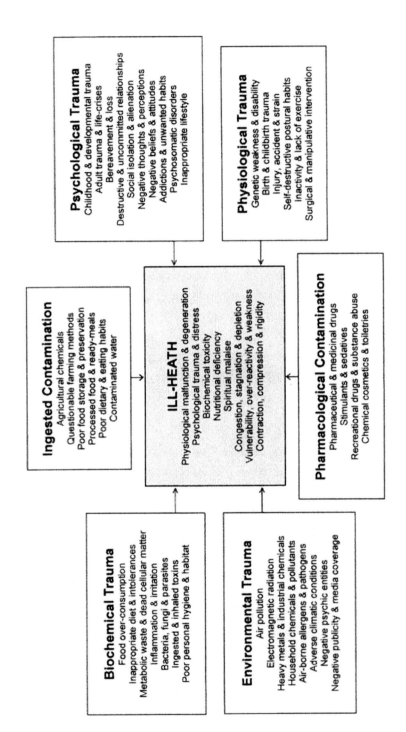

Figure 1.1 – *Where might your client's ill-health originate?*

Your client's genetic defects and her inherited disorders will be the obvious candidates for your attention but you may neglect to appreciate that she will, also, possess a given constitutional and metabolic type. Once you know what you are dealing with in terms of inherited factors, other conditions that are brought to your client's notice, in the guise of presenting symptoms, can be largely overcome or resolved, in some way, by identifying and treating the originating cause.

Ask yourself . . .

Does your client have any known and obviously inherited weaknesses or disorders? Does your client know of any genetic defects that must be continually supported and acknowledged yet she may be hoping that such conditions will simply go away? Has your client given up on her health issue because she believes that her condition must be genetic and would, therefore, be incurable? Does your client possess a robust and even impenetrable constitution? Does your client appear to be delicate, frail and weak by nature? Might your client have a naturally speedy or a sluggish metabolism that you can detect in her whole being? Could your client be tormented with the worry that she may pass on her genetic defects to her children? Can you identify any family traits in terms of your client's emotional and physical health? Does your client mistakenly believe that her inability to conceive can only be treated by surgical or drug-based intervention rather than by relieving her stress levels or rebalancing her endocrine system? Does your client with arthritis believe mistakenly that her state has developed because it runs in the family rather than being due to toxicity in her joints? Does your client firmly believe that she has a phobia of mice because her mother was frightened by one and had the same irrational fear?

What will be your client's physiological profile?

Your client may be able to tell you of any accidents or injuries that she has sustained but she may not be aware of other factors that will have done damage to her person. Your client may, for instance, dismiss birth trauma, childbirth trauma, life-threatening disease, minor physical strain and surgical intervention as just an inevitable part of life whereas, in reality, such invasion of the body will certainly have taken its toll. Your role may be to appreciate the impact that your client's adverse physical experience has had on her. Gentle verbal and/or physical probing, as appropriate, may be all that you will need to employ in order to become the ideal therapeutic sleuth with your client.

Ask yourself . . .

Does your client realize that her traumatic birth experience may have had a lasting effect on her ability to concentrate? Does your client appreciate that her blinding migraines may be the result of a partially-forgotten childhood injury? Could your client's chronic pain and immobility be due to subluxations of the spine that have impinged of the functioning of her delicate spinal nerves? Does your client have scar-tissue that might be acting as an impulse-generator that can upset the delicate electromagnetic fields within her system and its biosphere? Can your client consider that her childhood vaccinations have left their mark on her system and that the residue may need to be eliminated in order to prevent further damage? Does your client pay little or no attention to the fact that extensive dental work may have unhinged her entire skeletal system and caused untold malfunction? Can your client appreciate that major surgery or intensive medication has rendered her system highly toxic and functionally deranged? Does your client exhibit a serious malfunction in one of her vital organs that might be due to external stress of some kind? Will your client be accustomed to relying on harmful chemical medication in order to soothe her aches and pains? Can your client conceive that a physically abusive childhood has led to a whole catalogue of physiological and psychosomatic conditions? Does your client really believe that she has not suffered at all from a punishing regime of physical exercise accompanied by severe emotional stress? Does your client subscribe to a gentle and regular exercise regime? Might your client believe that she must be physically sound merely because she can walk about or can run fast? Will your client dismiss the fact that she has taken highly dangerous drugs that may have upset the whole balance of her biochemistry? Does your client consider herself to be in good health when, in reality, she will be in denial about the extent of her physical decline?

What will be your client's psychological profile?

All healing processes will require that your client undergo some form of emotional release and unconsciously-enlightening change. Your client will, in most cases of ill-health, need to address some form of underlying emotional issue that will usually date back to early childhood and will have had a knock-on effect into the present. Your client, for example, may have suffered stress or trauma during her developmental years and this will have impacted on her attitudes, her motivations and her perception all of which may be unhelpful and/or destructive to her. Adverse experience, in any walk of life, will, almost certainly, have an impact on your client. The best-case scenario may be merely that your client will have to contend with the regrettable knowledge that she is unwell and that her road to recovery may be a bleak prospect.

Ask yourself . . .

Does your client believe that the panic attack that she experienced last week was the result of an overcrowded supermarket rather than being due to a lifetime of worry? Does your client believe that her depressive melancholy stems solely from the fact that her partner walked out last month rather than being due to unresolved grief over her mother's death? Might your client have been the recipient of tough love during her formative years? Does your client tend to play down the fact that she had a violent or an abusive childhood and does she negate its enduring effect? Does your client feel inclined to blame the world for her troubles rather than addressing them full on herself? Could your client be over-interested in the wellbeing of the universe by way of deflecting herself from dealing with her own psychological issues? Will your client be prepared to acknowledge that her healing journey might need to encompass a thorough investigation of her emotional issues both past and present? Can your client acknowledge that her emotional distress will have an impact on those around her? Can your client appreciate that her roadblocks to recovery could be easily removed if she were to truly get in touch with her emotional life? Might your client be beset by negative thoughts and perceptions that can paint a dismal picture in her mind and could hold her back from moving forward? Could your client be impeded by a dead-weight in her emotional life? Can your client see any ray of light on the horizon that would give her hope of future recovery and success?

What will be your client's biochemical profile?

Often your client will be cruising along though life blissfully unaware of the dangers of environmental pollution, an inappropriate diet, dietary deficiency, over-consumption of poor quality food and a cocktail of medication and/or recreational drugs. Toxicity may invade the human system from the environment and/or be ingested, knowingly or otherwise, to such an extent that your client's system can no longer cope with the strain of defending itself. This build-up of toxicity will overload your client's system that will, consequently, begin to show signs of strain in the form of disease, vulnerability to infection, intolerance and degeneration. Your therapeutic discipline, therefore, may well need to embrace some knowledge of what is good and what is bad for the body and to gently convey this information to your client.

Ask yourself . . .

Would your client be unable to appreciate that fresh organic produce that may take a little time to prepare could be the answer to most of her minor ailments? Can your client appreciate that a diet of ready-made meals snatched in haste has rendered her in a state of malnutrition? Does your client think nothing of eating processed foods that are laced with harmful additives and preservatives? Does your client need to appreciate the fact that she has a serious mineral deficiency? Might your client simply be unable to assimilate the food that she eats efficiently enough for her system to be well nourished? Does your client have a chronic dysbiosis problem that might, in itself, be responsible for her ill-health or her lack of vitality? Has the poor condition of your client's intestinal flora opened the floodgates to systemic infection? Does your client suffer from a serious hormonal deficiency or an imbalance as a result of toxic invasion, a parasitic infestation or a post-viral syndrome? Does your client believe that nothing can be done for her digestive disorder yet she persists in eating the wrong kinds of food? Has your client's immune system been seriously impaired by her persistent intake of foods to which she is utterly intolerant? Does your overweight client suppose that she should not be eating fats when, in fact, she may merely be consuming the wrong kinds of fats? Does your client blithely dive for the medicine chest at the slightest provocation? Does your client treat her body as if it were a machine to be fixed by a mechanic and, thus, she takes no personal responsibility for what she puts into it? Has your client's metabolism slowed down to a snail's pace? Could your client even conceive of the fact that a total meta-

bolic cleansing and detoxification program would eliminate virtually all her long-term illnesses and disorders?

What will be your client's environmental profile?

Usually the immediate environment will be that part of modern living over which your client will have the least control. Your client may, therefore, at best, only be able to mount a damage-limitation exercise with regard to environmental pollution.

If your client lives in town, then, she will be exposed to city air, to overcrowding and to traffic emissions. In the country, your client may, similarly, be affected by air-borne allergens, by crop-spraying and by the use of agricultural chemicals. There can be no escape in the home either because of chemical cleaning agents, paint fumes and furniture preservatives that will pollute the very air that your client will breathe. Moreover, your client may relish in indulging in body pampering, may live a hectic life-style or be affected by adverse climatic conditions. Your client's living environment, and any stress that may result from lifestyle or habitat disharmony, will, furthermore, impact greatly on her health picture and her peace of mind.

The best hope may be simply for you to encourage your client gently to adopt a healthier lifestyle, as far as humanly possible, and not to compound her troubles by spending precious hours worrying too much about potential environmental problems. For your client with severe intolerances to certain air-borne substances, then, of course, she should seriously consider reducing her direct exposure to such irritants until the problem has been cleared or, at least, been contained to tolerable levels.

Ask yourself . . .

Does your client feel that her heart condition must be due to a lack of exercise rather than to an impaired cholesterol metabolism that came about because of living in a polluted environment? Might your client be in love with perfumes, soaps, cosmetics and other pampering agents that appear to give her a false sense of security? Does your client have trouble with a given internal organ because of some form of dental stress that might be affecting the acupuncture meridian-path associated with that organ? Could your client ever conceive that her mercury-amalgam dental fillings may well have seeped into her system and caused havoc?

Has your client's system been unknowingly invaded by heavy metals or other industrial pollutants that are causing untold damage? Does your client with numerous allergies and intolerances persist in exposing herself to these major irritants? Can your client appreciate that previous exposure to harmful pollutants may have contributed to her present health dilemma and weakened her immune system? Can your client find a convenient way of reducing her exposure to severely toxic agents? Has your client been the subject of ongoing geopathic stress that has resulted from strong magnetic fields generated by underground waterways or by disturbed land-masses? Might your client be continually exposed to electromagnetic stress from electrical equipment in her home or her office that could have adversely unbalanced the functioning of her body? Does your client live in a total muddle that will be reflected in her illness and her pessimistic outlook? Does your client wonder why she is unhappy and yet she might be living in a less than harmonious environment with inappropriate people? Does your client feel that her intimate partner should conform exclusively to her lifestyle and her conduct? Could your client be on the right path in life or will she be way off course?

What will be your client's pathological profile?

Your client's disease history may need to be studied in some depth in order to appreciate the way in which her ill-health has struck and what impact any pathological disorders may have had on her current state. As an alternative practitioner, you would not normally aim to treat symptoms but it may be that your client's current complaints could provide a key to the starting place for your investigation. You may, of course, find that a symptom that has already been given a label by a medical practitioner can allow you to gain an understanding of the nature of your client's suffering. Often long-term patterns can throw up information about the state of your client's health in terms of the type of infection or disorder to which she may fall prey.

Ask yourself . . .

What are the obvious and less obvious patterns that underlie your client's mind-and-body pathology? Could your client be beset with an over-reactive system that falls victim to every circulating germ? Has your client suffered for most of her life from a debilitating condition that manifested early in childhood? Does your client exhibit any repeating patterns in terms of her susceptibility to disease? What are the fungi and parasites in your client's world and how does she cope with these invaders? Has your client fed and hosted parasites of every description all her life? Might your client be over-burdened and be cluttered up physiologically and psychologically with infection, disease and malaise? Might your client be convinced that she has a serious and an untreatable condition because of erroneous public-domain knowledge? Will a knowledge of your client's disease history provide any clue to the way in which you might tackle her case? Could your client be crippled by an ongoing condition that she cannot seem to resolve unaided? Can you detect a link between your client's ailments and her emotional state or her spiritual self-awareness? Could your client's emotional wellbeing be dragged down by the knowledge of her illness or her susceptibility to disease? Should your client consider clearing her underlying infections before ever attempting to deal with her overt symptoms? Has your client's condition been given an unhelpful label by another practitioner?

Let's take an example – Cicero's story

Cicero worked as a naturopath but he harbored the usual assortment of concerns about his abilities and competence. Cicero felt that he was not good enough to be in practice, that he had insufficient knowledge to help his client and that other practitioners were more accomplished. Cicero, also, feared that he would lose concentration when working with his client because he was, generally, too disorganized to run his business. Furthermore, Cicero could detect himself becoming bored and disenchanted with the one-size-fits-all approach to treating his client.

Cicero decided to tackle his problems by continual personal and professional development that led him to extend his field of knowledge and expertise. Cicero, therefore, found himself constantly reading up on a vast array of related therapeutic topics and enquiring into issues, such as diet, nutrition, genetics, disease patterns and psychology, in order to take a more eclectic approach to his work. This new-found breadth of knowledge gave Cicero the self-confidence he needed in order to forge ahead with his practice. Cicero, also, elected to offer diagnostic analysis and health-checks to his client as means of providing himself with a competitive edge. On a more practical level, Cicero decided to off-load his paperwork on to an assistant and to update his accounting system in order to streamline his tedious office administration. This ploy had the added advantage of allowing Cicero to focus wholeheartedly on the comprehensive treatment of his client.

What would your client be aiming for?

Will there be such a thing as perfection and can it ever be attained by your client? Your client, as a human animal, can virtually never avoid the onslaught of life's pollution, toxicity and trauma both internal and external that will constantly pose a threat to her health. The sad fact may be that only a very small number of your clients will appear to be dedicated to doing everything possible to overcome these toxic obstacles. The best you can hope for, therefore, may be that your client will, at least, be trying, in some measure, to make the grade or be employing a damage-limitation exercise as a defensive regime.

What will be possible for your client?

In terms of recovery from malaise, it might be wise for your client to make the zenith her master rather than her slave because, in the proverbial ideal world, she should be aiming for nothing less than perfection. Despite the fact that a dizzy height can never normally be attained, this knowledge should not deter your client from aiming at the superlative because anything less would be a cop-out on her part.

Certainly you can encourage and reassure your client that a complete recovery should be achievable provided that she plays her part – assuming, of course, that this attainment would, in reality, be feasible in her particular case. If your client aims high, the results are likely to be surprisingly good. If your client elects to do nothing and merely to let things slide, because she believes that the ultimate cannot be fully realized, this could be regarded as a rather defeatist stance on her part. It would, of course, be best for your client to do all in her power to limit the extent of the damage and the decay as a means of motivating herself towards optimal health without paying too much attention to the ultimate outcome. At the very least, your client should be adopting a prevention-is-better-than-cure regime.

What will your client essentially achieve?

Mind-body-spirit detoxification and regeneration will endeavor to neutralize, to eliminate and to transform adverse agents and conditions in order to restore your client's homeostatic state of equilibrium (see Figure 1.2 – *How might your client attain optimal health?*).

Via the route of cleansing, toning, rebuilding, restoring, balancing and maintaining, your client can acquire optimal health, increased energy, more stamina, better mental clarity, longevity, vitality and rejuvenation as well as developing greater contentment, inspiration and creativity. For your client, this voyage may, of course, entail temporary withdrawal and/or permanent abstention from a given noxious substance in the interests of restoring and maintaining her improved health picture. The solution may be for your client to recognize and acknowledge, to overcome and resolve and, then, to move on in order to rebuild and to redevelop her life. As a practitioner, you can frequently take a god's-eye view of the situation and observe your client cleansing both past and present by tracing her patterns back and by recognizing the way in which former experience has been merely a composite of the daunting present.

Addressing one area in your client's life will, of course, have a knock-on effect into others and will culminate in improvements all around for her. Dealing with your client's emotional distress will, for example, resolve her unwanted habits, her inappropriate behavior and her physical ailments. Overcoming nutritional deficiencies will, in turn, release your client's pent-up emotions. Defeating traumatic anguish will, moreover, lead your client to greater contentment and to better social relationships. All therapeutic investigation will, by some means, bring about a degree of personal harmony, contentment, fulfillment and realization of your client's life purpose. Whatever your focus as an alternative practitioner, you will inevitably notice improvements in completely different areas of concern when treating your client within your own discipline.

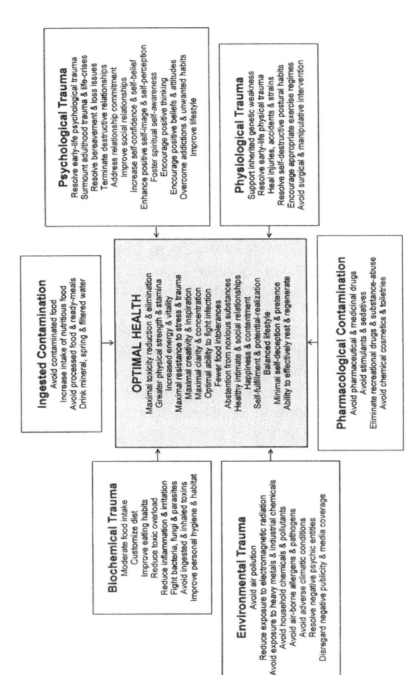

Psychological Trauma
Resolve early-life psychological trauma
Surmount adulthood trauma & life-crises
Resolve bereavement & loss issues
Terminate destructive relationships
Address relationship commitment
Improve social relationships
Increase self-confidence & self-belief
Enhance positive self-image & self-perception
Foster spiritual self-awareness
Encourage positive thinking
Encourage positive beliefs & attitudes
Overcome addictions & unwanted habits
Improve lifestyle

Physiological Trauma
Support inherited genetic weakness
Resolve early-life physical trauma
Heal injuries, accidents & strains
Resolve self-destructive postural habits
Encourage appropriate exercise regimes
Avoid surgical & manipulative intervention

Ingested Contamination
Avoid contaminated food
Increase intake of nutritious food
Avoid processed food & ready-meals
Drink mineral, spring & filtered water

OPTIMAL HEALTH
Maximal toxicity reduction & elimination
Greater physical strength & stamina
Increased energy & vitality
Maximal resistance to stress & trauma
Maximal creativity & inspiration
Maximal clarity & concentration
Optimal ability to fight infection
Fewer food intolerances
Abstention from noxious substances
Healthy intimate & social relationships
Happiness & contentment
Self-fulfilment & potential-realization
Balanced lifestyle
Minimal self-deception & pretence
Ability to effectively rest & regenerate

Pharmacological Contamination
Avoid pharmaceutical & medicinal drugs
Avoid stimulants & sedatives
Eliminate recreational drugs & substance-abuse
Avoid chemical cosmetics & toiletries

Biochemical Trauma
Moderate food intake
Customize diet
Improve eating habits
Reduce toxic overload
Reduce inflammation & irritation
Fight bacteria, fungi & parasites
Avoid ingested & inhaled toxins
Improve personal hygiene & habitat

Environmental Trauma
Avoid air pollution
Reduce exposure to electromagnetic radiation
Avoid exposure to heavy metals & industrial chemicals
Avoid household chemicals & pollutants
Avoid air-borne allergens & pathogens
Avoid adverse climatic conditions
Resolve negative psychic entities
Disregard negative publicity & media coverage

Figure 1.2 – *How might your client attain optimal health?*

Let's take an example – Quince's story

Quince works as a nutritionist, kinesiologist and iridologist who had clocked up many years of experience in his field. Quince's client complained of extreme lethargy that had reached the stage whereby she had become extremely unwell and virtually unable to function in her day-to-day existence.

Quince, first, tested his client in order to estimate where he would need to focus his attention initially when treating her. Quince's preliminary diagnosis indicated that his client would need to clear systemic candida as well as rectifying the effects of her leaky-gut syndrome. Following his diagnosis, Quince asked his client to undertake a metabolic clearing program over a protracted period of time to which she readily agreed. This lengthy biochemical cleanse, however, failed to bring about any expected results for his client. Quince's client did not feel any better and his diagnostic methodology continued to indicate toxicity within her system.

Next Quince decided to assess his client with a series of hair-mineral analysis tests and he discovered that her principal problem, even after her metabolic cleanse, was that uranium was present in her system in significant quantities. Quince, now, questioned his client carefully in order to determine how such a dangerous heavy metal could have invaded her body. It, then, transpired that Quince's client had lived abroad for some years only a short distance away from a weapons-testing plant. From this point on, Quince was, then, able to map out a tailor-made treatment-program that could deal with his client's underlying problem and could assist her in restoring her health to full capacity.

Let's take an example – Egeon's story

Egeon offers his clients a range of therapeutic skills that includes emotional-freedom therapy, eye-movement desensitization and reprocessing and neurolinguistic programming. Egeon's client sought therapy for a serious alcohol addiction, panic attacks and general dissatisfaction with life. Egeon's client was, also, interested in starting an astrology business but she lacked the motivation to get going on this project.

Egeon initially worked with his client in order to help her to resolve her major emotional issues in connection with her distress and, after some cathartic improvement, she began to get her life back on track once she was free of her addiction. Egeon's client, therefore, agreed to implement a goal-setting project whereby she would seek some part-time work as a short-term, stop-gap measure while she was in the process of setting up her astrology business.

At her next session, however, Egeon's client reported that she was despondent about implementing her plan and considered this to be a major setback. Further investigation revealed that Egeon's client had learned to associate success and the media-spotlight with a desire to panic and to escape from life. This revelation allowed Egeon's client to recognize the way in which she was avoiding involvement in life and why she hated the idea of earning a living or of being successful. This eye-opener enabled Egeon's client to understand her life more fully in context and to appreciate the way in which she was demotivated. The tables, now, began to turn for Egeon's client who immediately began to shift her life around by getting a part-time job and giving some astrology readings long before the agreed scheduled dates in her goal-setting strategic plan.

Egeon could, now, stand back and see clearly for himself the way in which his client's life had come to a standstill. Egeon could appreciate that his client's past traumatic experience, the emotion that this experience could generate, and the resulting symptomatic fear-based condition, were all part of a closely-knit triangle. Egeon, thus, began to understand that by breaking one aspect of the triangle, his client would, in time, be able to dissolve all her repeating patterns and her symptoms. Egeon was, also, interested to note that his client mentioned that her life had changed in a very casual manner because her addiction and her lack of motivation were not, now, issues that any longer worried her or hampered her progress in life.

2 WHAT WOULD CONSTITUTE ALTERNATIVE THERAPY?

What would be the premise of alternative therapy?

Will your client ever really appreciate the inestimable value of alternative therapy? It may be of vital importance for you to fully realize the way in which alternative therapeutic practice can help your client, irrespective of whether she may be a newcomer to the notion or a seasoned and dedicated exponent.

What will be the orthodox route?

The ultimate catastrophe of healthcare provision, in the so-called modern world, stems from the fact that the vast majority of people have come to live unquestioningly with the misguided notion that the system that already exists must be the best one. The man in the street usually regards alternative therapy as a quack-remedy and has been schooled in the doctrine that if you are ill you must take a pill. Mr Average relies on being told by some ill-equipped authority-figure that there must be something wrong with him and, then, would expect that the powers that be will decide how to put it right. If your client goes down this route, she will, of course, be handing over her brain lock, stock and barrel to someone else in the mistaken belief that the oracle must know best. A nice and easy solution if your client wishes to be absolved of all personal responsibility for her own healing process.

Western medicine will attack its patient's nasty and irritating symptoms without giving a fig for the root cause of any disorder and will regard the sick person as a collection of unrelated parts as if she were a mechanical device. The bottom line may be that the orthodox medical professionals, industrious and earnest as they may be, have maintained a tight citadel with the we-know-best-about-what-is-good-for-you mentality and this regime will encourage the don't-ask-any-questions mindset. Orthodox medical philosophy will have its own specially written rule-book. This modus operandi consists of specialization, compartmentalization of thinking, instilling fear in patients, categorizing symptoms, naming diseases, attacking bugs, pandering to the drug barons, using high-tech equipment and cutting out the offenders. The mainstream route, moreover, will, also, treat natural occurrences and processes as if they were dangerous activities and, therefore, they should be controlled in a clinical setting. The top-soil, however, will not be the garden. Perhaps the medical profession has relied too heavily on the philosophy of believing one's elders and betters.

Eastern philosophy, on the other hand, goes a long way towards meeting the needs of the sick and to align itself with alternative thinking. Eastern medicine, for instance, has the advantage of recognizing the holistic perspective and of incorporating regular meditative practice and spiritual awareness into remedial treatment.

Ideally, alternative practice could utilize the combined philosophies of both east and west in order to present alternative medicine as an integrated whole and to widely publicize its efficacy. What might need to happen, now, would be to bring alternative therapy as a free-standing entity into the limelight and to afford it center stage. Alternative practice could stand on its own feet by drawing on the scientific approach of the west and the spiritual orientation of the east. Perhaps the only viable way of establishing alternative therapy in its own right would be by allowing it to stand with one foot in both camps.

It may be difficult to bat for the minority but, perhaps, by reading this book you will further enlighten yourself and will truly appreciate your essential role in the scheme of things as an alternative practitioner by doing your tiny bit for the health of your client.

What will be the alternative route?

There can be no greater wisdom than that housed within the human system and its innate intelligence can constantly prove a ripe source into which you and your client can readily tap.

The natural route to recovery will activate your client's self-healing mechanism because this innate ability has been an inherent part of man's survival since the inception of the human race. This inherent self-correcting mechanism will be that part of your client to which you can speak when treating her. Your aim will be to enhance, to stimulate, to regulate and to support this self-balancing facility within your client so that her organism can get on with its job most effectively.

Natural therapy will aim to treat the root cause of your client's disorder rather than the surface-level symptoms. By the time symptoms have manifested and become troublesome, the originating cause of your client's malady will be firmly entrenched. Any attempt to regard your client's symptoms as the essence of her ill-health will be nothing less than short-sightedness yet most of the world do wallow in this misguided doctrine. The most vital ingredient for optimal health will be the cleansing of your client's mind, body and spirit of any phenomena that have invaded it during her lifetime, together with any inherited residue from personal and ancestral cellular memory. In whichever alternative realm you operate, you will notice that by merely focusing on one aspect of your multi-faceted client, this route will mysteriously lead her to additional benefit and relief in other parts of her intricate holographic being and life arena.

If you work principally as a body-oriented practitioner, you will inevitably watch your client undergo her emotional unfolding. Body detoxification will entail eliminating accumulated toxins, balancing bodily functions and making good any deficiencies in order to enable your client's physical and biochemical being to function efficiently. This process will, furthermore, of course, clear your client's mind of any disquiet and disharmony.

If you work from a mind-oriented standpoint, you will observe your client's physical ailments gradually beginning to diminish or even to disappear. Mind detoxification will involve your client in facing up to and resolving her emotional denial, her traumatic suppression and her negative programming in order to eliminate the backlog of her emotional and spiritual pain resulting from her life's stress and trauma. This course of action will, consequently, enhance your client's physical wellbeing as well as uplifting her spirit and enriching her outlook.

Let's take an example – Lysander's story

Lysander works as a nutritionist who has chosen to specialize in the treatment of cancer patients. Lysander was approached by a cancer sufferer who wished to explore an alternative means of curing her liver cancer because of the dismal prognosis that she had been given. When Lysander's client arrived for treatment, he explained, in principle, what his methodology would entail. Lysander's client had been informed by her conventional medical practitioners that she was, now, a terminal case and had, consequently, been granted a place in a hospice for the remainder of her days. Lysander's client had, previously, undergone extensive chemotherapy and had, recently, been operated on in order to place a stent tube in her liver with the aim of unblocking her bile duct and, thus, maintaining some degree of her liver function.

Lysander treated his client over a period of several months and her progress was rapid and successful. Once his client had recovered fully, her medical practitioners were keenly interested in the methods that Lysander had, so successfully, employed and were full of praise for both client and practitioner. When Lysander's client had fully recovered, moreover, her surgeon elected to remove her stent tube because he was convinced that her liver could, now, function adequately and unaided by this mechanical device. Lysander's client was, subsequently, admitted to hospital and her operation to remove the stent tube was successful. Regretfully, however, Lysander's client contracted the methicillin-resistant staphylococcus aureus (MRSA) viral infection from which she died in a matter of days while still in hospital recovering from her operation.

What will be the healing-crisis phenomenon?

All forms of detoxification and rebalancing of your client's system at the root-cause level will bring about the inevitable healing crisis that has been so maligned by the critics of alternative practice and so dreaded by those on the receiving end (see Figure 2.1 – *How might the healing crisis assist your client?*).

The healing-crisis phenomenon will simply be your client's innate self-correcting wisdom at work in earnest. Any change, for the good, will disturb and will aggravate your client's organism in order to generate a better outcome or an improved state. Moreover, your client may need to revisit some portion of her personal history that will have involved mental, emotional, physical and/or spiritual trauma in order to unwind the damage that she has sustained back in the past.

Only by comprehending and accepting the inevitability of her healing process can your client ever hope to remain optimistic while on that important, yet tumultuous, road towards resolution and recovery. The healing-crisis phenomenon will, of course, be a knotty little problem for your uninitiated client to grasp under any circumstances. Your client may subscribe to several commonly-held misconceptions and, in addition, she may not wish to accept the validity of the it-gets-worse-before-it-gets-better phenomenon when she finds herself in the middle of a healing experience wherein the going is extremely tough.

It will, naturally, be vital for you to explain to your client the significance of her healing crises and the importance of staying the course when any do occur. Disaster will, without doubt, strike if your client regards any healing reaction as if it were a symptom ripe for suppression. For your client to suppress or to ignore her healing reaction may be a mistake easily made in the climate of popular fallacies about the way in which the mind and body heals itself and in the light of propaganda from the mainstream camp. As a practitioner, of course, you may be so familiar with the healing-crisis phenomenon that you can often neglect to tell your client until it could be too late.

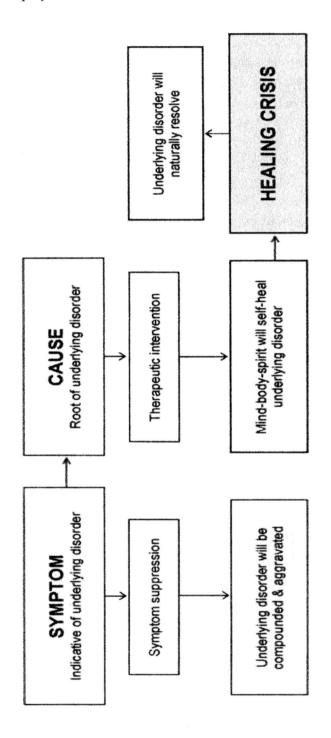

Figure 2.1 – *How might the healing crisis assist your client?*

Let's look at it another way – Clearing out the cobwebs

One day you wake up and notice that there sits a spider's web on your window sill. Oh dear, you think, I must clear the cobwebs from my dwelling place. So you set to with pan and brush in order to rid yourself of this annoying and this dust-collecting impediment to your happiness. Once you have done your housework, you can, then, rest easy at nights. You retire to bed proud of your house-keeping skills and dedicated to domestic-goddess perfectionism.

When you open your eyes the next morning, however, your sweet dreams are shattered. Right there is the offending cobweb back again to haunt you. Damnation! So, once more, you don the maid's cap and the rubber gloves and thoroughly dust away the unwanted cobweb in order to ensure that you will continue to sleep peacefully and can retain that virtuous feeling of being house-proud and conscientious. The pattern, however, may repeat itself for several days – the virtue of doing your housework and, then, having your peace devastated the next morning when the felonious spider has worked industriously overnight and has returned to plague you. Life may become a nightmare for you. You may even begin to dream of spiders and, then, develop arachnophobia.

Your existence will become more intolerable until, at long last, you discover the truth about the spider and the spider's web. No amount of war-waging on the accursed cobweb will be effective, of course, because the spider's web is not the spider. The cobweb cannot, simultaneously, be the manufacturer of the cobweb. The sad fact remains that the web will only disappear from your domain after you have chased the spider from your house and he has taken up permanent residence elsewhere. Was this a painful learning-curve for you even though it might have been one that will ensure your permanent freedom from those confounded cobwebs in the future?

Let's take an example – Viola's story

Viola had qualified as a hypnotherapist but was, however, slow to get her practice going because deep down she believed that she did not have the necessary experience in order to handle any disturbing or difficult cases. Viola, in consequence, invested widely in additional training in order to broaden her knowledge-base and to perfect her skills. Viola, then, began tentatively to set up her practice but, of course, still looked for evidence of her success via her clients.

Viola's breakthrough came when she was helping her client to over-come the trauma of rape. Viola's client had discussed her traumatic experience at length in therapy but she still felt that there was something incomplete because she had not had an opportunity to bring her assail-ant to justice. Viola's client, also, confessed that her traumatic experience had robbed her of her ability to feel sane and to interact normally with men. Viola, now, had to think on her feet in order to help her client to resolve her misery. Viola decided that her client might need to address her rapist verbally and to say what she really felt. Viola was, thus, able to uti-lize a gestalt technique whereby her client was invited to imagine that her rapist was in the consulting room and that she could, now, tell him what she really thought of him. In amazement, Viola listened as her client, then, spilled out an unending flow of her deep-seated thoughts and her overwhelming emotions. Viola felt privileged to witness this unfolding of her client's repressed thoughts and emotions that were finally coming to the surface in an unbridled stream.

After this break-through session, Viola's client felt that an enormous weight had, at last, been lifted from her shoulders and that she, then, believed herself to be liberated in order to live a full life again. Viola, too, felt released by her creative handling of her client's case and discovered a new-found confidence. Following this experience, Viola, consequently, realized that she would, in fact, be able to deal with any demanding cases and to offer her client a wide range of creative techniques in the future.

Where would alternative therapy be right now?

Will you comprehend where your client may stand in the alternative equation? The whole premise of alternative method-ology will be that of identifying and of resolving the underlying root cause of your client's disorder rather than attempting to treat and/or to suppress her symptoms. Staunch critics will maintain that the alternative system has its healing-crisis inconveniences and cost-factor limitations but such opponents often, also, ne-glect to appreciate the inherent restrictions and drawbacks to orthodox medical philosophy.

What will alternative therapy achieve?

The principal benefit of employing alternative therapy will be that your client's treatment will endeavor to bring about a lasting relief from her physical, her psychological, her biochemical and her spiritual malaise. Under the alternative umbrella, therefore, your client will be treated holistically rather than as a collection of disparate parts. A complete cure, therefore, may, given time and patience, be a more realistic goal for your client with alternative practice than with the drastic approaches taken by the allopathic disciplines. In contrast to allopathic medicine, however, the alternative profession may not be the quick-fix route or even the least painful direction for your client to take. A complete recovery, when possible, may, however, bring to your client many painful healing reactions that will require her to be endowed with dogged determination and teeth-gritting tenacity.

Where will practical reality sit for you?

As an alternative practitioner, you may, in many respects, need to work cheek by jowl with conventional practice or, at least, to take into consideration your client's experience within the medical or surgical arena. In a utopian world, your client will have managed to evade orthodox treatment totally and, thus, will not have been manipulated, operated on, vaccinated, received radiography or taken any chemical drugs. Ideally, your client will, also, not have been exposed to junk-food, to environmental pollutants, to recreational stimulants, to physical injury, to emotional stress or to any unfriendly media. But, alas, Utopia will be far from reality and, if it were, you would be out of business anyway.

Your client, in many cases, may have elected to or, of necessity, been compelled to partake of the conventional approach of western medicine, perhaps, as a surgical life-saving measure or in a medical emergency. Whether working alternatively, or in a complementary manner, within the orthodox caring profession, you will, doubtless, be confronted with many clients whose previous history, cultural programming and current concepts will, invariably, have embraced allopathic thinking and fast-lane living.

You may, therefore, find yourself caught up in the mainstream system by default when treating your client and you may feel as if you are being sucked into, or, possibly, even straightjacketed by, conventional medical approaches. At some point in your career, as a result, you may need to seriously consider to what extent you would be willing to work alongside one or more orthodox medical practitioners. On the one hand, you might regard yourself solely as an alternative practitioner and, thus, would not wish to treat any client who is seriously wedded to conventional practice. On the other hand, you may feel quite at home as a complementary practitioner and be perfectly able to work in conjunction with your client's general medical practitioner or her specialist.

Ask yourself . . .

Would you prefer to be a truly alternative practitioner or do you see yourself as a complementary therapist? Can you predict where your client might be coming from in terms of her opinion of orthodox medical practice and intervention? To what extent has your client been exposed to, been harmed by or been interfered with by orthodox medical practice? Has your client benefited at all from her surgical or her drug intervention? Can you take your client's forays into conventional practice into account when treating her condition? Do you need to gently return your client to the medical profession because she may, now, be beyond your help? Can you work within your client's parameters as a complementary practitioner? Has your client been exposed to a lifetime of negative programming in favor of conventional medical practice? Does your client automatically assume that if she is feeling ill, she should consult a doctor? Has your client been using orthodox methodology as a means of evading her underlying issues?

Let's take an example – Portia's story

Portia had qualified as a reflexologist and had achieved an impressive track-record in this healing profession in which she believed implicitly. Because of her dedication in this field, Portia found herself attracted to a new and exciting branch of work, entitled neuroflexology, that addresses her client's self-healing mechanism via her nervous system. As with any new form of treatment, Portia sought verification and validation of the ground-breaking work that she was undertaking in order to support her sound faith and conviction about its efficacy.

Portia was privileged one day to meet a client who was crippled with arthritis due to a motorbike accident that had occurred some 45 years ago. Since this accident, Portia's client had never been able to walk properly and had been in and out of hospital for several surgical operations including a recent hip-joint replacement operation. Portia administered treatment to her client and awaited the results. Portia was, then, fascinated to observe the self-healing pattern that her client adopted. Portia's client exhibited no immediate responses during her treatment but between her sessions she somehow found a means of activating her self-healing, self-regulating and rebalancing mechanisms. Portia's client, thus, returned for subsequent sessions with remarkable results merely because the nerves of her upper and her lower body were activated and harmonized to beneficial effect. By this means, Portia was able to offer others concrete proof of the efficacy of this revolutionary practice.

How would your client view alternative practice?

Will your client ever truly appreciate why alternative therapy can be so effective? You will benefit greatly from recognizing your client's stance on alternative practice and by gauging her knowledge and her appreciation of your particular therapeutic angle. When you know what your client believes, it will give you a head-start when treating her and will enable you to assess her chances of ultimate success.

What will be your client's perspective on alternative methodology?

You may find it advantageous to determine your client's opinion of, and her attitude towards, the alternative realm in order to understand her mindset in terms of her ability to recover. It could be useful for you to consider your client's opinion about which therapeutic practices may be appropriate for her. It would be advisable for you, for instance, to note the types of alternative therapy and medical intervention that your client might regard as being beneficial.

You can, in this way, glean insight into where your client may be coming from and, consequently, where she might be going on the road towards recovery. From this angle, you may be able to assess your client's chances of success and her willingness to comply with the somewhat rigorous and off-the-wall dictates of your alternative practice. If your client proves to be seriously wedded to the orthodox medical view of illness, however, it may be an ordeal for her to adjust to your methodology and to your philosophy. Sometimes your client can be subtly educated but, on other occasions, she may just be a lost cause.

Ask yourself . . .

Can you gauge your client's attitude and opinion of the efficacy of alternative therapy? Does your client really understand and truly believe in the principles of alternative medicine? Why has your client chosen to seek the alternative route? Could your client's thinking still be very much entrenched in orthodox methodology and this appears to limit her appreciation of the alternative route? Will your client be in the dark ages when it comes to appreciating alternative methods of healing? Does your client fully comprehend the fact that the alternative route may not be the straightforward, quick-fix option? Might your client be undertaking a number of alternative therapies simultaneously and this could indicate that she has signed the pledge of recovery from declining health, excessive stress and discontentment? Will your client be a newcomer to your form of alternative therapy but, nevertheless, can greet the experience with an open mind? Could your client be curious to discover the benefits of alternative therapy?

Let's take an example – Edgar's story

When Edgar first became a shiatsu practitioner, he had not really bargained for the healing qualities that might be inherent in bodywork. One of Edgar's first clients came into his consulting room and, as soon as he began to massage her, she began to cry uncontrollably. Edgar was slightly disconcerted by his client's tears because he felt that her reaction was interrupting his work. Edgar was, of course, appreciative of the fact that his client was in distress and that she needed to unload and, so, he encouraged her to talk about the nature of her problems. Edgar's client confessed to a feeling of loneliness having been seriously rejected by her mother. Edgar received this news with empathy because it reflected his own personal experience but decided that he should proceed with the massage for which his client was paying.

On reflection and discussion with his supervisor, Edgar realized that he was quite at liberty to allow his client to talk and that it might have been immaterial to her whether he actually completed his therapeutic massage. At her next session, Edgar's client reported that she had re-

ceived an enormous amount of relief from her tears and that she had gained as much from talking and being able to express her feelings as she did from receiving her massage. Edgar had, thus, learned an important lesson. It was not what he did but who he was that mattered when it came to treating his client and some moderate deviation within a session might be quite acceptable when it is, in fact, what she requires from her practitioner.

Let's take an example – Bernardo's story

Bernardo practices dietary therapy and naturopathy and has acquired a reputation for being able to handle serious, life-threatening cases. Bernardo greeted his new client who informed him that he had been diagnosed with leukemia and wanted to explore the possibility of taking the alternative route towards recovery because he had been given an extremely poor prognosis from his mainstream medical practitioners. Bernardo's client was able to appreciate that alternative medicine could provide a recovery prognosis and believed himself to be prepared for any necessary hard work in order to overcome his condition.

Bernardo initially devoted much time to explaining, in detail, to his client precisely what would be involved in taking the alternative route towards recovery. Bernardo emphasized that alternative methods of treating cancer might need to involve some major detoxification procedures, fasting and colonic irrigation as well as demanding many dietary and lifestyle changes – to say nothing of addressing important psychological issues. Bernardo, also, mentioned that, in order to effect a complete recovery, his therapeutic procedures would probably need to take place over an extensive period of time but at his client's own acceptable pace.

At this news, Bernardo's client exclaimed that he had, essentially, not bargained for having to undergo what he considered to be such a rigorous regime. Bernardo's client protested that he had hoped that he could merely be given some nutritional supplements in order to combat his disease. Bernardo, then, reiterated the fact that his client's serious condition, that may have been building up for several decades, will, of necessity, require some pretty drastic measures before it can be conquered. Bernardo's client, however, still agreed to proceed with his therapy believing that he could, in fact, take the pace because the ultimate goal would be very worthwhile.

Bernardo used a bioresonance system at his client's first session in order to identify the starting-point for his treatment. Bernardo, also, prescribed some nutritional supplements that would stimulate his client's immune system. When Bernardo's client returned for his next session, he reported, with some degree of disappointment, that his condition had not improved. Bernardo, once again, explained to his client that the alternative route cannot be a quick-fix regime and listed the reasons why. Prior to his next appointment, however, Bernardo's client rang to cancel his scheduled session and announced his intention to return to blood transfusions and the conventional route. Bernardo's client had, now, gained an appreciation of what might be involved in alternative medicine but had, somehow, finally decided that he would not play this card and would resign himself to his inevitable fate.

How would your client view her overall health picture?

Will your client really be able to see it like it is? Your client's attitude to her own health and its implications will be the starting-block from which she can, fundamentally, progress. Whether you are dealing with your client's physical, psychological, biochemical, mental and/or spiritual health, the jumping-off point will be for you to decipher the way in which she views herself and her health picture.

How will your client regard her own health prospects?

The extent to which your client will be willing to embrace alternative methodology will have a direct impact on her health and her recovery prospects. Often your client's beliefs and convictions about the efficacy of alternative practice will be the key to her ultimate success. A firm belief in and appreciation of alternative practice may be all that will be needed in order to imbue your client with the courage to pull herself through.

If your client can be open-minded and versatile in her thinking, your job may be more straightforward and rewarding. If, however, your client greets you with precious little experience of previous therapy, or any form of alternative practice, then, this may be an indication of where she sits on the road to success. If your client has entertained many years of ill-health, and yet has failed to recover using any allopathic means, you may need to have a clear view of her attitude to her own health problem in order to meet her halfway along the street. Ultimately, it must be your client's responsibility to do the work of self-healing under the alternative umbrella and her attitude in this respect may spell either failure or success, accordingly, for her.

Ask yourself . . .

Will your client be fully dedicated to the whole philosophy of alternative medicine? Will your client be aware of everything that she may be required to accomplish and any sacrifices that she may need to make in order to attain satisfaction? Could your client be firmly entrenched in the allopathic camp and merely making a gesture towards alternative practice as a last-ditch desperate resort? Could your client be partially or wholeheartedly skeptical about the therapeutic discipline that you practice and will her disbelief affect her progress? Could your client ever appreciate that her symptoms will indicate that her innate intelligence may be doing its vital healing work? Does your client regard her symptoms, or her healing reactions, merely as a nuisance and a definite sign that she must be getting worse? Does your client need to have any faith in the remedies or the supplements that you intend to prescribe? Is your client optimistic about her chances of a full recovery?

Will your client's personal healing journey be tough?

If your client has been steadfastly glued to the philosophies of orthodox medical intervention, her road may be steep and an uphill struggle in the field of alternative practice. Medical interventionist theory will foster quick-fix thinking in your client, coupled with a drug-taking mindset. Your client, moreover, may not have been exposed to the notion that she has any personal responsibility for her own recovery process. Your client may, also, find the concept that her symptoms are not the originating cause of her disorder to be a very strange pill to swallow. Often these deeply entrenched beliefs will stem from the I-must-do-what-authority-figures-tell-me outlook that may have colored your client's unquestionable wisdom for many decades.

If your client maintains an unrealistic approach to her condition and her symptoms, she may fail to appreciate that what she

41

regards as an unpleasant indicator of malaise will, in fact, be evidence of the beneficial healing crisis. When your client sheds tears, for example, she will be unwinding the misery of the past in order to unshackle herself and to move on. If your client complains of aches and pains, she may be cleansing and detoxifying her organism. If your client needs to sleep for days on end, her system may be taking the initiative and getting on with the healing process.

It may be advisable for you to think long and hard about your client and to attempt to get into her mind on the question of therapeutic intervention. This ploy may be a means of arming yourself with the knowledge of how you could tackle your client's case. You may need to provide your client with much information and a few lively pep-talks before she can make an informed decision about her own health prospects. The main purpose of this exercise will be to take the heat off you and to place the responsibility where it should sit – squarely on your client's shoulders.

Ask yourself . . .

Does your client possess the necessary mental attitude to stay the course with dedication and perseverance? Has your client taken on board the concept of the inevitable healing crisis and its likely consequences for her? Does your client appear dedicated to the task in hand or could she be only vaguely interested in her process of recovery? Can your client suspend her disbelief and her need to find logical answers to all her problems? Will your client be prepared to see through her own recovery or does she still expect the proverbial quick-fix from you? Will your client be doing everything that she can in order to bring about her own success in therapy? In what ways might your client be hindering her own progress? Would your client be at all interested in her health as her long-term dedication to wellbeing and longevity or does she simply want to feel better right now? Does your client have any evidence to support the fact that she may be attempting to bring herself to a state of optimal good health?

Why would your client choose your therapy?

Will you discover your client's unique starting-block? Your first consideration may be an appraisal of your client's healing voyage within the alternative profession to date and the reasons why she has finally landed on your doorstep.

Will your client have done her homework about you?

Your client, in an ideal world, will attend your clinic because she fervently believes that what you might have to offer will work for her. Your client, however, will have her own agenda for choosing you and your therapeutic discipline but her motivation may be far from the ideal. Your client will, in essence, need to have a full appreciation of the particular brand of therapy that you have to offer and the way in which it could be of assistance to her. If your client does not seem to be clued up in this respect, the outcome for her may be disappointing. It will, however, be a dangerous game to take on the responsibility for your client's decision-making process because her choice to consult you should be hers alone.

Your client, in many cases, will choose a therapeutic methodology according to the type of symptoms that she will exhibit. If your client suffers with physical pain or from bodily discomfort, she may select a bodyworker because she believes the methods employed will rectify her physical ailments and her somatic malfunctions. If your client has been beset with bereavement issues or with relationship problems, she may seek a counselor or a psychotherapist. If your client has digestive disorders or any allergic tendencies, she may consult a nutritionist, a homeopath or a herbalist. If your client suffers from psychic distress or from spiritual malaise, she may track down a spiritual healer or a spiritual psychotherapist because she will be drawn to metaphysical philosophy. In all these cases, your client will have made something of an informed choice as a conscious, mental process.

If your client has been recommended to you by a successful predecessor who has publicized your services enthusiastically, she will certainly be on the right foot. Your new client, however, may not necessarily possess the exemplary ingredients for victory that your former client might have had in great abundance. Your potential client, of course, may merely make a random choice and may not really know, at all, why she has chosen to consult you. Your client may simply have waggled a pin around which landed on your name. You may, thus, find yourself taking a gamble and you may, by chance, pull it off because your client, coincidentally, will have what it takes to make it work. If your new client might really not be very self-aware or, in essence, be too naïve about the healing process, she may be totally unsuited for your methods of practice simply because she has not done her research thoroughly enough.

Ask yourself . . .

What, if anything, does your client know about you and your therapeutic discipline? Has your client made an informed choice about coming to see you? What factors have led to your client's decision to visit you? Has your client tracked you down like an enthusiastic blood-hound because she has been convinced that you are the ace for her and that no-one else will do? Does your client have a clear picture in her mind of what your treatment will entail and the way in which it can help her? Has your client been recommended to you by an enthusiastic exponent of your methodology? Does your client simply trust the universe to send her to the right person and will not really need to take any significant part in the decision-making process? Would your client be a suitable candidate for your particular brand of alternative therapy? Does your client possess a totally unrealistic notion of the therapy that you offer because of what she has seen on the television or heard from someone else who was, similarly, unenlightened? Could your client be seeking your practice as a last-ditch measure with no real conviction in her mind of the efficacy of the therapy that you practice? To what extent do you feel responsible for your client's choice of therapy and her practitioner?

3 WHERE WOULD YOU FIT INTO THE ALTERNATIVE PICTURE?

Where would you see yourself in the alternative therapy world?

Will you know where you reside in the therapeutic universe? Any practitioner working in the alternative field should not be working in a vacuum and wearing a blindfold. For this reason, it will be of enormous value for you to have, at least, an appreciation, if not a viable working knowledge, of the scope of the principal therapies in the alternative realm (see Figure 3.1 – *What might constitute alternative therapeutic practice?*).

This chapter will not be meant to be a hard-hitting lesson in the various alternative and complementary practices but will be merely designed to broaden your perspective. If your interest has been stimulated by this information, then, it might be advisable for you to speak directly to one or more practitioners in your field of interest or to research these additional areas in your own way.

What else will happen in the alternative world?

It could be vitally important for you to recognize that you are a part of a whole spectrum of alternative practices all of which will seek the same ultimate aim – to help your client to activate

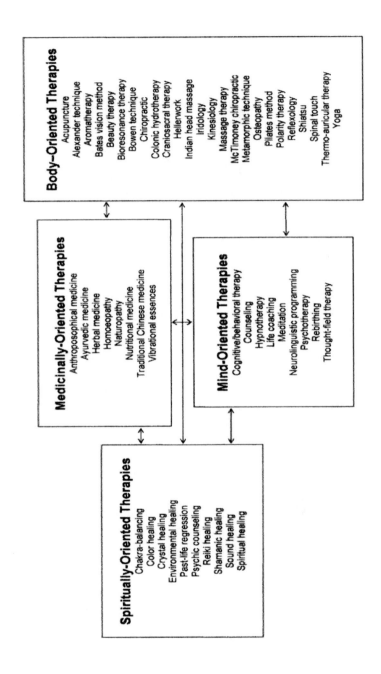

Figure 3.1 – *What might constitute alternative therapeutic practice?*

her self-healing mechanism that will, in turn, influence her mind, body and spirit.

Your client will be a unique being whose disorders or whose troubles will have had an all-encompassing impact on her and she may well need to partake of many different therapeutic disciplines in order to acquire the optimal health for which she might strive. You may, therefore, find it useful to understand all the facets of your client's healing journey and her mindset as an integrated picture. You should, also, have an appreciation of the effect and the impact of any other supporting treatment that your client may, simultaneously, be receiving as this knowledge will help you to understand her holographic picture more realistically. It can, therefore, be useful for you to view your particular therapy as a part of a whole range of therapeutic disciplines any of which may be chosen by your client. With this theme in mind, you could, now, consider the main therapeutic disciplines in the field of alternative therapy and complementary medicine in order to view yourself and your client within the therapeutic cosmos.

How will you find yourself in the alternative maze?

When defining your own therapeutic practice, the most vital point will be for you to realize that your specific contribution will have many resonances into related fields. Your work as an alternative therapist, therefore, will not be discrete and far from isolated. As an alternative practitioner, you will, quite justifiably, be affronted even at the suggestion that you or your practice could be packaged up and labeled. Indeed, it may well be utter folly to even attempt to compartmentalize any given holistic treatment because of the significant impact that one discipline will have on many other fields within the alternative arena. For the sake of convenience, however, the main alternative practices have been categorized here into pigeon-holes with the aim of allowing you to see where you might fit into the overall frame.

When considering your slot in the therapeutic universe you may wish to ponder the ways in which you might brush other areas of alternative practice when treating your client. If you are a psychologically-oriented practitioner, then, you will realize that psychosomatic healing will, also, result from your client's exploration of her inner mind. If you practice bodywork or you administer alternative medicines of any description, then, you will appreciate that, by implication, you will be helping your client with her emotional issues because her body will tell its own story. If you are a therapist in the spiritually-inclined domain, then, your client's healing will inevitably take place on many different levels of soul, mind and body.

Ask yourself . . .

Do you really have an appreciation of what your colleagues in other domains might set out to achieve? How many times have you made forays into distantly-related fields of alternative practice? Have you personally received a range of alternative treatments in order to improve your own health? Do you frequently exchange information and treatment sessions with other practitioners? Are you familiar with the ethos of bodywork and physically-oriented practice? Would you know what the philosophy of metaphysical practice constitutes? Have you investigated the premise of psychotherapeutic or counseling practice? Do you know why medicinally-oriented therapies can be so effective? Do you consider that your way must be the only workable solution to any problem that your client may exhibit?

What would constitute body-oriented therapy?

Will you understand the purpose of alternative physical medicine? The body-oriented practitioner will, principally, take a hands-on approach to his client and, in doing so, will activate and encourage her self-healing mechanism from a physical standpoint (see Figure 3.2 – *What might be an overview of body-oriented therapy?*).

Acupuncture

Aims To stimulate and regulate the flow of qi energy through the body's meridian-channels; to expand or reduce energy-centers along the body's midline; to adhere to the principles of traditional Chinese medicine.

Methodology Inserting and manipulating very fine needles into the body's acupoints; applying heat, pressure, friction, suction or impulses of electromagnetic energy to the acupoints.

Related approaches Auricular acupuncture, do-in, shiatsu, thought-field therapy, toyohari, tuina therapy, zero-balancing.

Alexander technique

Aims To promote ease of movement, flexibility and effortless functioning; to restore natural postural balance; to reduce muscular tension and eliminate unnecessary strain; to reduce compression and alleviate pain.

Methodology Reeducating the mind and body using a gentle hands-on approach.

Related approaches Feldenkrais method, Hellerwork, medau movement, Norris technique, Trager work.

Aromatherapy

Aims To improve and maintain physical, mental and emotional health; to encourage lymphatic drainage; to alleviate stress and adverse health disorders.

Methodology Applying plant-derived essential oils to the skin for systemic absorption using massage techniques.

Related approaches Beauty therapy, massage therapy.

Bates vision method

Aims To improve defective vision and relieve eye-strain.

Methodology Reeducating the mind in order to resolve the emotional impact of impaired vision.

Beauty therapy

Aims To enhance natural beauty, relieve stress and protect the body against environmental pollutants.

Methodology Applying a range of holistic personal care treatments to the skin and body.

Related approaches Aromatherapy, massage therapy.

Bioresonance therapy

Aims To treat disease, overcome allergic reactions and eliminate bodily toxins.

Methodology Employing a computerized device in order to detect and balance electromagnetic energy frequencies within the body.

Related approaches Biofeedback therapy, light therapy, radionic therapy, skenar therapy.

Bowen technique

Aims To release tension and resolve energetic blockage within the body's musculature and connective tissue; to restore bodily balance, promote healing potential and initiate detoxification.

Methodology Applying precise, light and gentle movements to specific areas of the body.

Related approaches Spinal touch therapy.

Chiropractic

Aims To maintain the structural health and functioning of the spine and nervous system; to restore a full range of movement and relieve pain.

Methodology Utilizing neuromusculoskeletal manipulation, mobilization and adjustments to soft tissue.

Related approaches Diaphragmatic release, McTimoney chiropractic.

Colonic hydrotherapy/Colonic irrigation

Aims To stimulate the release of stored faecal matter from the colon; to enhance the eliminative performance and function of the bowel; to implant herbal or probiotic preparations into the colon.

Methodology Introducing purified water into the colon under pressure and employing massage techniques in order to expel faecal matter.

Craniosacral therapy

Aims To enhance the quality of cerebrospinal fluid and promote self-healing on a systemic and cellular level.

Methodology Utilizing gentle palpation techniques in order to reflect and focus on areas of trauma within the system; stimulating the self-healing mechanism in order resolve traumatic stress.

Related approaches Cranial osteopathy, metamorphic technique, spinal touch.

Hellerwork

Aims To unblock restrictive structural patterns from body-memory; to correct postural alignment; to access and resolve emotional-holding patterns.

Methodology Combining deep-tissue massage, movement education and verbal dialogue.

Related approaches Rolfing.

Indian head massage/Indian champissage

Aims To relieve accumulated bodily tension; to stimulate circulation; to restore joint movement; to improve hair condition.

Methodology Employing Ayurvedic massage techniques to the upper body.

Iridology

Aims To determine holistic health, levels of inflammation and the extent of systemic toxicity; to identify genetic predispositions and gauge the efficiency of the body's eliminative organs.

Methodology Examining the iris, pupil and sclera of the eye using magnifying devices.

Kinesiology

Aims To realign the musculo-skeletal system; to restore emotional balance; to reestablish biochemical functioning; to determine the body's dietary and nutritional requirements.

Methodology Employing energetic muscle-testing, detecting movement imbalances and utilizing verbal questioning.

Related approaches Allergy testing, holographic repatterning.

Massage therapy/Swedish massage

Aims To improve general wellbeing; to stimulate the body's energy flow; to induce the breakdown of tissue adhesions.

Methodology Stroking and kneading the body's soft tissue.

Related approaches Amna, aromatherapy, Aston patterning, Ayurvedic massage, baby massage, biodynamic massage, chavutti thirumal, holistic massage, hot stone massage, kahuna bodywork, manual lymphatic drainage, remedial massage, shiatsu massage, sports massage, thalassotherapy, Thai yoga massage.

McTimoney chiropractic

Aims To relieve muscular strain within the body.

Methodology Identifying and correcting subtle imbalances in the system; changing the tension surrounding the joints and interacting with the natural elasticity of tendons.

Related approaches Chiropractic.

Metamorphic technique
Aims To transform self-limiting patterns held within the body.
Methodology Applying a light touch on spinal reflexes in the feet, hands and head.
Related approaches Craniosacral therapy, spinal touch.

Osteopathy
Aims To return the musculoskeletal system to normal alignment and proper integration; to rectify structural abnormalities and restore healthy functioning; to positively influence any malfunctioning internal organs.
Methodology Employing techniques of manipulation, stretching, articulation and massage.
Related approaches Cranial osteopathy, craniosacral therapy, massage therapy, osteomyology, physiotherapy, skeletal balancing, zero-balancing.

Pilates method
Aims To strengthen the body's core postural muscles; to develop balanced alignment; to improve posture, coordinated movement and stamina; to aid concentration and breathing.
Methodology Utilizing slow, controlled movements combined with breathing techniques.
Related approaches Alexander technique, Norris technique, breathwork.

Polarity therapy
Aims To ensure the uninterrupted flow of bodily energy between various polar opposites.
Methodology Treating the body as a vibrational energy field with a neutral center between a positive and a negative electrically-charged pole.
Related approaches Ayurvedic medicine, Chinese medicine, Pilates method, yoga.

Reflexology
Aims To stimulate energy flow; to encourage toxic elimination; to initiate cellular repair within the body.
Methodology Massaging precise reflex areas on the feet and hands that correspond to specific regions of the body.
Related approaches Massage therapy, metamorphic technique, neuro-flexology, reflex-zone therapy.

Shiatsu/Acupressure
Aims To encourage the body to eliminate toxins; to improve the flow and quality of qi energy through the meridian-channels.
Methodology Utilizing a combination of massage pressure and stretching techniques.
Related approaches Acupuncture, do-in, tsubo therapy, tuina therapy, Zen shiatsu.

Spinal touch
Aims To restore the body's natural structural balance in order to maintain health.
Methodology Applying a light touch to the body in order to realign the center of gravity to the sacrum.
Related approaches Craniosacral therapy.

Thermo-auricular therapy/Hopi ear candles therapy
Aims To heal energy depletion or imbalance within the body.
Methodology Inserting a hollow cotton tube impregnated with honey and herbs into the ear; igniting the tube in order to produce gentle stimulating warmth.

Yoga
Aims To acquire dynamic balance and integration of the mind, body and spirit; to induce relaxation and engender self-awareness; to improve posture and maintain healthy bodily functioning.
Methodology Employing postural exercise combined with breathing and concentration techniques.
Related approaches Aston patterning, Pilates method, qigong, t'ai chi ch'uan.

Figure 3.2 – *What might be an overview of body-oriented therapy?*

What will body-oriented therapy embrace?

The body-oriented practitioner will usually make physical contact with his client in order to manipulate, to persuade, to stimulate, to encourage and/or to reeducate her physical vehicle. If you are a bodyworker, you will, of course, be acutely aware of the fact that in making direct contact with your client's physical being, you will, also, be making an intimate connection with her biochemistry, her spirituality and her emotional responses to past injury, trauma or malfunction.

Physical contact may involve your client in either dramatic or subtle manipulation as with chiropractic, Hellerwork, massage therapy, osteopathy and reflexology. Light-touch therapy for your client may, conversely, include the Bowen technique, craniosacral therapy, the metamorphic technique, polarity therapy and spinal touch therapy whereby physical intervention will be either minimal or virtually non-existent. Your client may, also, be tenderly persuaded to reeducate her own physicality using the Alexander technique and the Bates vision method.

The subtle energy fields of your client's meridian-channels and energy-centers may be encouraged to rebalance and to regulate in order to increase or to decrease the flow of her life-force energy using acupuncture, thermo-auricular therapy and shiatsu methodology. Other interventionist therapeutic disciplines that your client may elect to undertake might include beauty therapy, colonic hydrotherapy and Indian head massage.

Diagnostic therapies that are often used in conjunction with natural physical medicine will include bioresonance therapy, iridology and kinesiology all of which are non-interventionist methods designed to establish your client's state of health with a view to treatment.

Practices, such as the Pilates method and yoga, have, also, been included in the category of body-oriented healing work as a vehicle for coordinating your client's physical movement with her spiritual wellbeing.

Let's take an example – Philostrate's story

Philostrate trained as a craniosacral therapist and, in the process of undertaking his training, he found that he benefited enormously both from practical work with fellow-trainees and from the personal therapy that he received in order to support his learning. By this means, Philostrate managed to overcome a long-standing illness that had been labeled as largely untreatable by the orthodox medical profession.

Philostrate found that he benefited from processing his physical and his emotional baggage in numerous ways both during and after his training and this, in turn, had a positive effect on his subsequent work as a practitioner. Philostrate's personal healing journey had the effect of making him more grounded and in touch with the peace and stillness within himself. Philostrate's newly-discovered inner peace, consequently, enabled him to become more sensitive to the needs of others, more perceptive and better able to work from the heart with his client. Philostrate's personal experience of therapy, also, made him more aware of his own boundaries and those of his client. From a sound place, therefore, Philostrate quickly learned to establish safety, openness and presence with his client. Philostrate eventually found himself able to deal with any difficult client with equanimity and with compassion and to remain non-judgmental when pushed into a tight corner.

Philostrate spent much time in building up his personal resources in order to equip himself with the skills to maintain a practice in an exacting field of operation. Being better resourced through personal therapy, supervision and the support of his colleagues, also, meant that Philostrate grew stronger both for himself and for the benefit of his client. Philostrate, thus, became both a well-rounded practitioner and a contented person who became very fulfilled in his work.

What would constitute medicinally-oriented therapy?

Will you realize the profound potential of natural alternative medicine? The practitioner of alternative medicine will prescribe supplements, remedies and preparations for his client and, in doing so, will give her body and its biochemistry a helping hand in order to facilitate natural healing (see Figure 3.3 – *What might be an overview of medicinally-oriented therapy?*).

Anthroposophical medicine
Aims To harmonize the spiritual self and the physical body using natural remedies.
Methodology Reviewing and adjusting lifestyle, diet, constitution and natural biorhythms.

Ayurvedic medicine
Aims To improve the force and quality of bodily energy.
Methodology Interpreting diagnostic and constitutional criteria; providing dietary guidelines and suggesting lifestyle changes; utilizing herbal inter-

vention and detoxification procedures.

Herbal medicine/Phytotherapy/Botanical medicine
Aims To rebalance the body's biochemical reactions.
Methodology Administering herbal preparations derived from natural plants and plant-products that possess therapeutic, medicinal, aromatic and savory qualities.
Related approaches Kanpo, tissue-salt remedies.

Homeopathy
Aims To stimulate inherent healing energy within the body at a cellular level; to facilitate the body's beneficial healing crises and strengthen the recovery process.
Methodology Exploiting the properties of naturally-occurring plant, animal or mineral remedies by healing like with like.
Related approaches Allergy testing, vibrational essences, tissue-salt remedies.

Naturopathy
Aims To stimulate the body's natural healing mechanism; to attain a state of detoxification; to improve resistance to disease and sustainable equilibrium.
Methodology Reviewing and adjusting disharmonious lifestyle habits.
Related approaches Dietary therapy, herbalism, hydrotherapy, light therapy, magnotherapy, nutrition, ozone therapy, tissue-salt remedies.

Nutritional medicine
Aims To aid detoxification and eliminate toxic build up; to promote the assimilation of nutrients and reestablish biochemical efficiency; to overcome food intolerances; to assist the body to heal from specific diseases.
Methodology Providing dietary guidelines and suggesting lifestyle changes; prescribing nutritional supplements and natural remedies.
Related approaches Allergy testing, Ayurvedic medicine, biorhythm theory, chelation therapy, dietary therapy, glandular therapy, magnotherapy, metabolic typing, naturopathy, orthomolecular therapy.

Traditional Chinese medicine
Aims To regulate the flow of qi energy through the body's meridian-channels.
Methodology Providing remedial medication, pharmacology, herbal remedies and nutritional guidance; administering acupuncture, massage and

qigong as an integrative practice.
Related approaches Acupuncture, herbal medicine.

Vibrational essences

Aims To restore mental and emotional balance and induce holistic self-awareness; to rebalance any negative emotions that underpin disease and malfunction.

Methodology Utilizing the healing potential of plants and flowers.

Related approaches Animal essences, gem essences, healing herbs, homeopathy, light essences, radionic therapy, shell essences, star essences, tree essences.

Figure 3.3 – *What might be an overview of medicinally-oriented therapy?*

What will medicinally-oriented therapy embrace?

The medicinally-oriented practitioner will administer natural supplements and remedies obtained from the plant kingdom and the natural world in order to treat his client's ailments. If you utilize alternative medicinal preparations, you will appreciate that your client will need to address her physiology, her psychology and her spirituality and her energetic biosphere as a means of treating any specific disease pattern or any adverse condition.

Alternative medicine for your client may include age-old practices, such as Ayurvedic medicine and traditional Chinese medicine, as the flagships of ancient cultures as well as embracing the western equivalent in the guise of Anthroposophical medicine and its accompanying lifestyle philosophy. Nutritional medicine might constitute the big-guns approaches to your client's holistic medical treatment in that nutritional supplements claim to be the natural basis of many allopathic drugs and, therefore, can have a dramatic impact on her biochemistry. Natural approaches to healing that your client may, also, consider might include herbal medicine and naturopathy. More subtle, yet extremely powerful, forms of energetic medicine for your client will include homeopathy and vibrational essences. These approaches to natural healing will address imbalances and malaise in the subtle energy fields that govern the functioning of your client's system.

Let's take an example – Jessica's story

Jessica worked as a medical herbalist but she decided to supplement her practice by gaining an additional qualification in craniosacral therapy. Once qualified, Jessica found that her therapeutic practice began to take a new direction when she had expanded her compass of expertise.

With herbal medicine, Jessica was accustomed to taking a thorough case history but, yet, she did not venture too far into the psychological aspects of her client's case. After Jessica had gained her qualification in craniosacral therapy, she found that her client was more inclined to experience emotional release during treatment but she was somewhat at a loss to know how to handle this aspect of her newly-acquired skill. Jessica's dilemma centered on whether she should combine her two disciplines, whether she should spend more time counseling her client at the conclusion of a session and to what extent she should conduct an in-depth case study into both her medical and her emotional history.

As her experience developed, Jessica found a means of combining her skills and knowledge in order to treat her client more effectively. Jessica elected, invariably, to take an in-depth case history as well as combining her therapies when the occasion arose and when her client was in full agreement. Moreover, Jessica was able to hone her counseling skills and she intuitively learned when to intercede and when to remain silent with her client. This strategy, therefore, allowed Jessica's client to unload emotional baggage, as and when necessary, and at a pace with which both parties could admirably cope.

What would constitute mind-oriented therapy?

Will you appreciate the dynamic power of psychological resolution? The practitioner of psychological medicine will facilitate his client in unraveling her emotional, her motivational and her behavioral disorders that have led her to experience unpleasant symptoms and to exhibit negative behavioral traits (see Figure 3.4 – *What might be an overview of mind-oriented therapy?*).

Cognitive/behavioral therapy
Aims To restructure negative attitudes and beliefs; to encourage realistic perception; to overcome maladaptive behavior and undesirable habits.
Methodology Resolving emotional problems and relationship difficulties;

overcoming habitual behaviors and lifestyle complications; reshaping negative perception.

Related approaches Biofeedback therapy, brief solution-focused therapy, cognitive-analytical therapy, laughter therapy, personal-construct therapy, rational-emotive behavior therapy, reality therapy, stress management.

Counseling

Aims To resolve emotional difficulties; to conquer unwanted habit disorders; to overcome social dysfunction and lifestyle problems.

Methodology Encouraging self-reflection and facilitating perception-alteration.

Related approaches Analytical and creative transformation, hypnotherapy, gestalt therapy, psychotherapy.

Hypnotherapy

Aims To resolve emotional disorders and relationship difficulties; to overcome negative behavioral patterns; to stimulate motivation.

Methodology Inducing a relaxed state in which the mind's resources can be accessed in order to transform the root cause of a disorder.

Related approaches Analytical and creative transformation, autogenic training, counseling, guided imagery therapy, journey work, meditation, stress management.

Life coaching

Aims To achieve important life goals; to facilitate sustainable lifestyle changes.

Methodology Clarifying needs; seizing self-growth opportunities and exploring aspirations.

Related approaches Cognitive/behavioral therapy, fearless life coaching, the Silva method, stress management.

Meditation

Aims To bring about overall relaxation; to foster self-enlightenment, healing and spiritual development.

Methodology Encouraging the quietening of a busy mind by narrowing the focus of attention on the experience of the moment; observing the flow of experiences, mental images and physical sensations.

Related approaches Hypnotherapy, yoga.

Neurolinguistic programming
Aims To accomplish a desirable outcome by overcoming impediments to motivation.
Methodology Enhancing sensory awareness and cultivating a flexible attitude of mind.
Related approaches Cognitive/behavioral therapy, time-line therapy.

Psychotherapy
Aims To resolve psychological distress and maladaptive behavior.
Methodology Employing verbal techniques and unconscious communication; identifying symbolic behavior and reeducating the mind; utilizing psychoanalytic, humanistic, transpersonal and integrative techniques in order to gain insight into the workings of the mind.
Related approaches Analytical and creative transformation, art therapy, augenblick therapy, bioenergetic analysis, cognitive/behavioral therapy, counseling, drama therapy, dance-movement therapy, dream therapy, gestalt therapy, Hellerwork, Hoffman process, hypnotherapy, music therapy, play therapy, psychology, psychosynthesis, Shen therapy, voice therapy.

Rebirthing
Aims To release emotional blockages; to alter outmoded life patterns; to foster empowering self-awareness.
Methodology Facilitating conscious and connected breathing techniques and focused awareness.
Related approaches Breathwork, holotrophic release, Shen therapy, spiritual healing.

Thought-field therapy/Emotional freedom technique
Aims To release energy blockages from the body; to relieve emotional stress and disturbing thought patterns; to resolve unwanted behavioral patterns.
Methodology Tapping the body's acupoints and stimulating the meridian-channels.
Related approaches Acupuncture, shiatsu.

Figure 3.4 – *What might be an overview of mind-oriented therapy?*

What will mind-oriented therapy embrace?

The practitioner of mind-oriented therapy will encourage his client to gain insight into her psychological disharmony, her adverse emotive reactions and any unwanted behaviors. If you are a practitioner in the psychological realm, you will realize that the power of the mind can be the key to your client's overall health picture in terms of her emotional state, her relationship issues, her enjoyment of life, her realization of potential, her susceptibility to ill-health and her physical degeneration.

Psychologically-oriented practice will include conventional methodologies, such as cognitive and behavioral disciplines, that endeavor to alter your client's mental and motivational processes by conscious intervention. This category of active psychological intervention for your client will, also, include the more recently-founded fields of life coaching and neurolinguistic programming. Under the umbrella of insight-oriented practice, can be found counseling, hypnotherapy, psychotherapy, rebirthing and thought-field therapy all of which will take a back-door route towards your client's psychological resolution by facilitating subtle unconscious change and enlightenment.

Let's take an example – Calpurnia's story

Calpurnia wanted to enter a profession in which she could really help people and, so, she chose to train as a humanistic counselor. Calpurnia, furthermore, wished to increase her own personal understanding and her self-awareness as part of her self-questioning approach to life in general. The training course that Calpurnia underwent allowed her to realize that her calling was probably making up for all those occasions, in the past, when she had been prevented from assisting others.

Calpurnia's initial fears about becoming a therapist centered on whether counseling would work for her client and how she might feel if this worry turned into a reality. Calpurnia was, also, concerned that she might do damage to her client or that she might exacerbate her disorder. Calpurnia, however, found a means of overcoming her predicament by researching into other methods of counseling, such as psychosynthesis, in order to broaden her field of understanding. Calpurnia was interested in investigating the effectiveness of related methods of treatment as a means of extending her toolbag of therapeutic interventions. In this

61

way, Calpurnia was able to safeguard herself somewhat against her own fears. Subsequent experience in the field, also, helped to increase her self-confidence as she progressed in her new career.

What would constitute spiritually-oriented therapy?

Will you have explored the significance of metaphysical philosophy? The spiritually-inclined healing practitioner will channel healing energies and will administer spiritual guidance to his client in order to assist her natural recovery from her emotional, her physical or her spiritual disharmony (see Figure 3.5 – *What might be an overview of spiritually-oriented therapy?*).

Chakra-balancing
Aims To balance the flow of energy within the body's principal energy-centers.
Methodology Employing energetic healing methods and verbal skills.
Related approaches Color healing, crystal healing, mediation, reiki healing, sound healing, spiritual healing.

Color healing
Aims To correct energetic imbalances within bodily systems and internal organs.
Methodology Identifying and utilizing color frequencies, light frequencies and vibrational energies.
Related approaches Aura soma, aurora therapy, crystal healing, gemstone healing.

Crystal healing
Aims To realign the system's chakras; to rebalance the energetic fields that encompass and surround the physical body.
Methodology Applying natural crystals and stones to the physical body and the immediate environment.
Related approaches Gemstone healing.

Environmental healing
Aims To eliminate harmful electromagnetic stress in the environment, the home and the workplace; to review and rearrange the living and working environment in order to create harmony and balance in accordance with ancient Chinese principles; to improve relationships, prosperity, health and

wellbeing.

Methodology Realigning and rechanneling earth energies; examining and creating an ideal living and working environment.

Related approaches Electromagnetic stress healing, feng shui, geomancy, geopathic stress healing, space clearing.

Past-life regression

Aims To relieve current stress and ill-health disorders that may have emanated from previous incarnations.

Methodology Facilitating the recollection and resolution of events from previous incarnations of the spirit.

Related approaches Psychic counseling, spiritual psychotherapy.

Psychic counseling/Spiritual psychotherapy

Aims To provide psychic guidance in order to assist healing and life-purpose fulfillment.

Methodology Facilitating mind exploration, dream counseling and past-life regression.

Related approaches Astrological counseling, clairvoyance, metaphysical therapy, spiritual psychotherapy.

Reiki healing

Aims To activate the system's natural healing ability.

Methodology Allowing the body to draw on and utilize the vital ki energy force from the universe.

Related approaches Aurora therapy, cellular healing, chakra-balancing, holographic repatterning, johrei, metaphysical therapy, radionic therapy, seichem, seiki solo, spiritual healing, vortex healing.

Shamanic healing

Aims To access, retrieve and heal traumatized parts of the soul.

Methodology Entering an altered state of consciousness in order to summon healing forces from the parallel universe.

Related approaches Illness extraction, past-life regression, sacred song, soul retrieval, spirit-power healing, spiritual prescriptions.

Sound healing

Aims To induce beneficial changes within the body and its electromagnetic field.

Methodology Employing a number of vibrational instruments in order to

heal the mind, body and spirit.
Related approaches Aurora therapy, music therapy.

Spiritual healing
Aims To repair and reestablish the body's auric energy field.
Methodology Channeling energy into the body either by the laying on of hands or remotely over distance.
Related approaches Aura cleansing, aura balancing, chakra-balancing, Kirlian photography, reiki healing, therapeutic touch.

Figure 3.5 – *What might be an overview of spiritually-oriented therapy?*

What will spiritually-oriented therapy embrace?

The spiritually-oriented practitioner will employ natural and readily-available healing energies in order to assist his client in recovering from any malaise in an endeavor to harmonize her spirit. If you are a practitioner who heals the spirit of your client, you will frequently address her transpersonal realm and will tap into her personal energy fields. As a spiritual healer, of any description, you may regard your client as a voyager through this life in order to facilitate her soul in its evolution and its fulfillment of her current life's unique purpose.

Spiritually-oriented therapy will often work, seemingly without any agenda, in order to achieve health improvement in your client as in the case of chakra-balancing, reiki healing and spiritual healing. This category, also, encompasses the healing domains in which colors, crystals, gemstones, lights, sounds and vibrations are utilized as the healing medium. With certain spiritual practices, such as past-life regression, psychic counseling and shamanism, your client will specifically and purposefully address her psychic evolution.

Feng shui, space clearing and geopathic stress clearance are, also, some prime examples of a practice in which your client will be encouraged to rearrange her immediate environment as a means of accessing the deeper recesses of her emotional wellbeing, her intrinsic motivations and her lifestyle harmony.

Let's take an example – Dionyza's story

Dionysa practices as a shamanic healer who regularly conducts healing groups and, also, teaches her work to groups of prospective healers. In conducting shamanic groups, Dionysa found that the main problem that a number of her clients, and her trainee practitioners, would experienced was the difficulty of facing the fact that healing comes from within the individual and not from an outside agent. Dionyza observed, for instance, that a given client might initially flee from a group workshop and / or indulge in blaming others for her own inability to make progress.

Dionyza noticed, consequently, that often the number of trainees on one of her practitioner training courses would diminish considerably as the training program progressed. Dionyza discovered, however, that once the heal-thyself notion had been realized by her client, it might be as if she had been hit with a bucket of cold water. Only when Dionyza's client had reached this realization could she, then, successfully continue with her therapy or with her training program. Dionyza, however, remained true to herself by offering compassion to her client, or her trainee, but not sympathy for those who were struggling with the notion of personal healing responsibility. Dionyza could merely provide the space in order to facilitate her client's self-help but could go no further until this awareness had dawned.

Dionyza's client, or her trainee, however, would frequently elect to return, at a later date, rather like a boomerang when she had fully appreciated her role in the equation of self-healing. By this time, either Dionyza's client had proved ready to undertake her healing program or her former trainee had, then, done enough self-investigation to be able to tackle her training course.

Where would you fit into the holographic framework?

Will you continually rediscover yourself anew? Pause for a moment, perhaps, in order to consider what you have just read. It may be wise for you to keep an open mind constantly about your therapeutic work, and to regularly reexamine your place in the alternative or complementary profession, in order to appreciate your unique role as a therapeutic practitioner.

How will you view yourself as a holistic practitioner?

By viewing your own therapeutic practice and those of your colleagues, consider, now, to what extent you can address your client's needs in terms of physical, psychological, biochemical or energetic therapy. Taking a long, hard look at yourself, your work and your place in the scheme of things can be an approach that you could regularly adopt, in the future, as a means of evolving yourself and expanding your horizons. A flexible approach will allow you to develop, if you wish, or simply to be yourself and remain content with your ability to get it right for yourself. This self-examination process may be the key to your professional unfolding and your self-development.

If you are a bodyworker, for example, you may consider that you work exclusively with your client's physicality or, alternatively, you may largely wish to embrace the energetic and the psychological fields within your work. If you are a practitioner who works with your client's biochemistry, you may elect to cater entirely for her medicinal needs but you could, in addition, have a strong leaning towards cures for physical ailments rather than mental and emotional malaise. If you are a talking-cure practitioner, you may work solely in the domain of your client's mind but, on the other hand, you may decide to veer strongly towards employing a spiritually-oriented practice. If you are a practitioner in the metaphysical field, you may, similarly, work largely with your client's bioenergies but you may, also, focus your practice on emotional healing or lifestyle guidance.

Ask yourself . . .

Can you see yourself differently, now, and do you feel that you know where you might fit into the healing picture? Have your views of your own practice altered, in any way, as result of your review of alternative therapies? Can you imagine yourself in the whole scheme of things from an alternative, a complementary and an allopathic viewpoint? Why not experiment with your concept of the alternative picture and where you might slot into the frame? Do you feel inclined to train in a new field or, at least, to find out more about another area? Do you regard yourself as part of a hologram, now, rather than working in isolation from related disciplines? Can you appreciate the work of your colleagues more realis-

tically and will this new-found knowledge assist your client? Could you undertake a self-examination quest in order to highlight those areas that you would regard as being your unique field of operation and those that you think apply exclusively to others? How might you reflect on your own practice differently in future once you have discovered yourself in the holographic alternative universe?

PART 2
YOU AND YOUR CLIENT

4 WHERE WOULD YOUR CLIENT BE COMING FROM?

Who would be your average client?

Will you expect your client to be as successful as you were when you jumped the fence? With the aid of wishful thinking, of course, it can be easy for you to imagine that you will be greeted by a whole stream of ideal clients. This precious notion, however, may not constitute reality in the therapeutic profession. More often than not, your average client will be encumbered with many imperfections and your job will often become more complex as a result.

Will your client share your enthusiasm?

When you undertook your own therapeutic journey, you may have been a gift to your practitioner but your own personal experience could tend to cloud your expectations of others. Your client, for instance, may not be as enthusiastic as you were when you undertook the same therapeutic process.

Despite an emphatically-expressed desire to change, your client may be inclined to put numerous barricades in her own way and to resist the therapeutic process with intense vigor. We do not live in an ideal world and your client may well be battling with years of unhealthy living and unwise cultural programming neither of which will be conducive to a healing mission in the alternative domain. Your client may still be hoping for the painless fix and may be only partially interested in self-improvement.

Your client may be more interested in her pottery workshops or in keeping her family entertained. Your client may be wholeheartedly resistant to the alternative approach – a stance that could be purely born out of blind terror or merely due to inadequate information. Your client, moreover, may simply be passing through in order to see whether what you might have to offer could be of any use to her. Worst still, you may never ever discover what your client's trip-up mechanisms actually might be.

Be not disheartened when you do not meet the perfect client every time you open your door. The totally-committed client can be a very rare beast. Coming to terms with this fact may be a part of the practical lesson that you will need to learn in order to survive personally and professionally in the business. Your reward of job-satisfaction may only come when you have swallowed this bitter pill.

Ask yourself . . .

Do you expect your client to be brimming with effusive enthusiasm? Perhaps you were the ideal client and you undertook your own personal therapy with dedication, zest and fervor and, now, wonder why the rest of the world does not follow suit? Do you expect every client to be the same as the first one you met or the last one you cured completely? Do you vainly hope that your client will approach your consulting room from the standpoint of a sound belief in the efficacy of your methodology? Do you want all your clients to be exemplary so that they will spread the good news to others? Can you capitalize on your client's willingness merely to hold on to the mast in a storm? Can you weed out any totally-disinterested clients and focus on those who are more dedicated to self-healing and recovery?

Would your client really comprehend your therapeutic approach?

Will your client really be a wise cookie? Your client may need to be able to appreciate the subtleties of your particular therapeutic approach in order to gain any true benefit from her therapy.

Will your client fully understand what you have to offer?

Your client may arrive on your doorstep with many unrealistic or several misguided notions about your practice none of which will be helpful to her progress. Occasionally, you may be able to dispel most of your client's outmoded notions about your therapeutic methodology but sometimes not. If your client has been ill-informed, or has not done her homework painstakingly, you may be faced with a mismatch in terms of what she expects and what you can, in fact, deliver. It would not, of course, be wise for you to compromise on what you are prepared to offer to your client. When you step outside your comfort-zone, and your personal-integrity realm, you could either put yourself out of your depth or merely diminish your job-satisfaction.

Ask yourself . . .

Does your client really understand what you have to offer or will she be laboring under a misguided impression? Can you easily expel any of your client's misconceptions about your practice methodology? Has your client watched too many television programs or read the wrong coffee-table literature? Are you ever tempted to offer your client what she might be demanding rather than sticking to your guns? Might you be trying to do the impossible with your client in the hope of pleasing her? Can you recognize why your client may not be fully committed to her healing process? Would you like the ride with your client always to be smooth, sunny and hassle-free? Do you definitely need to feel successful in order to create your personal illusionary peace of mind? Can you gently reeducate your client along the right path?

Let's take an example – Berowne's story

Berowne, an acupuncturist, began to treat his client for a long-standing candidiasis condition that was characteristically accompanied by depression and insomnia. At the first meeting with his client, Berowne discovered that she needed constant reassurance that he would be able to assist her with her condition. Berowne's client, for example, would repeatedly asked him "Do you think you can help me?" or "You are able to help me, aren't you?". Berowne's client seemed desperate for this guarantee because other more conventional methods of treatment had failed in the past.

Berowne was, however, able to take a realistic stance when his client asked these demanding questions. Berowne assured his client that he was capable of helping anyone but that the hard work would have to come from her. Berowne was steadfast in stating that his job was merely to be the catalyst and not the converter. Berowne, then, suggested to his client that she ask herself "Do I think I am capable of overcoming my troubles by getting in touch with the essence of my disorders?". If the answer to this question was in the affirmative, the next question that Berowne's client would need to pose might be "And do I feel that this practitioner could assist me?".

When these questions were posed by Berowne's client to herself, she, subsequently, began to take quite a different view of her condition and this change of perspective put a special complexion on the equation. The ball was, now, back in the court of Berowne's client who had to decide whether she wished to play tennis before receiving any accolade for success at the game. This challenging self-questioning, thus, led Berowne's client to consider some dietary and some lifestyle changes in addition to consulting her practitioner and endeavoring to overcome her debilitating disorders. Berowne had, therefore, rendered his client a great service by purely being true to himself.

Would your client be on the right track?

Will your client understand what she might need from you? Your client may ideally be an excellent candidate for the therapy that you have to offer and at which you may be an acknowledged expert. Alternatively, your client may be barking up the wrong tree entirely and really she ought to be visiting a different practitioner in another discipline altogether in order to address her disorder (see Figure 4.1 – *What might be your client's best healing option?*).

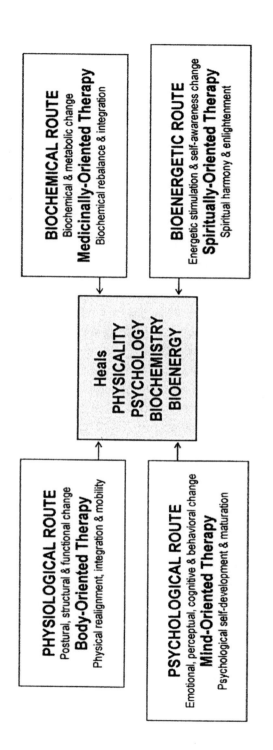

Figure 4.1 – *What might be your client's best healing option?*

Will your client be clued up about her healthcare?

You may need to carefully reflect on whether your client will be on the right track when she consults you and whether your professional expertise can assist her further in her quest. When you consider the ways in which your client may be attempting to help herself, you may often find that she has taken a somewhat ill-advised route. Your client, in reality, may be chasing the wrong kinds of rabbits and, then, wondering why the magic does not work. Your client may, also, have been searching relentlessly in the wrong quarters in the mistaken belief that the steps that she has been taking will inevitably deliver the goods. It could be that your client may be endeavoring to tackle her problems from the wrong angle even within the alternative field. Perhaps, for instance, your client might be dedicated to body-oriented therapy when, in fact, she should, simultaneously, be looking at her emotional health or her nutritional requirements or both.

Your client may, of course, have been previously wedded to the notion that allopathic medicine will hold the key to her success and she may have been inclined to take chemical drugs or to undergo risky surgery. Your client may have been accustomed to doing what she has been told by the medics who may be blinkered and uninformed with regard to her particular disorder. Your client may, at last, be making a detour into alternative practice but her heart may lie elsewhere. The question you must, now, ask yourself, therefore, might be whether she can reform.

It may well be that you will need to come to terms with your client's approach to her healthcare and not to interfere with her choice of methodology or her practitioner. Conversely, you may need to gently suggest to your client that there could be a different route that she might consider. Often you will be walking a tightrope when making a decision about whether to remain silent or else to intervene with your client's choices and her inclinations. Essentially, it must be your client's decision but some unbiased information from you may assist in her decision-making process. When indecision strikes, you could, possibly, discuss the question with your supervisor or with a mentor and, then, consider what might be in the best interests of your client in her particular circumstances.

The decision to refer your client to another alternative practitioner with a given specialism that will be outside your field of expertise should, of course, be a card that you can play when you feel, in any way, out of your depth. It will be no shame or any poor reflection on your ability as a practitioner to move your client gently in a different direction. You may, of course, suffer the dire consequences of any reluctance on your part to exercise this right of referral if you continue to flog the proverbial dead horse with your client. After referring your client to another practitioner, you may still be able to help her but in a more supportive role rather than being her principal agent of change.

Ask yourself . . .

Do you feel all at sea when attempting to assist your client to improve or to recover? Could your client's problem principally be of an emotional or a spiritual nature and will you simply be supporting her through a difficult time by providing your brand of alternative treatment? Does your client need to address her biochemical toxic stress in addition to investigating all her lifestyle issues that have contributed to her malaise? Does your client need to be spiritually cleansed as well as receiving her regular massage or her beauty treatment? Would your client be more responsive when in an environment where she can exploit her beliefs in psychic evolution or in reincarnation? Does your client need a more forceful form of treatment rather than your soft-touch approach? Would your client be better off with a gentle and non-invasive approach instead of your hefty handwork? Does your client really need to turn herself over to a surgeon or to go down the chemotherapy route in order to save her life? Has your client gone too far down the allopathic road for it to be possible for her to claw herself back by any alternative means? Does your client still believe that her high blood-pressure or her kidney stones cannot be cured? Does your client believe that her psoriasis must be an abnormal skin condition rather than a liver malfunction and consequent toxic overload? Might your client still be locked into the belief that, as a clinical practitioner, you can take her suffering away instantly? Has your client turned on the bath-water but forgotten to put in the plug?

Let's look at it another way – Making a birthday cake

A chef decides to make a delicious fruit cake for a special birthday party. The recipe for this celebration cake has been tried and tested over time. The usual procedure would be for the chef to begin by purchasing fruit, nuts, butter, sugar, eggs, flour, spices and brandy. The ingredients would, then, need to be mixed together and, after that, the mixture must be baked in an oven for a given period of time. Decorative icing could, next, be applied to the cake after it has been left to cool. Once the cake has been fully decorated, it can, thus, be enjoyed with relish at the birthday party.

If, however, the chef considers that, for some reason, it may be better to begin to make the cake by boiling some cabbage, and he will not deviate from this course of action, then, of course, a fruit cake will not be the final result. The chef may boil cabbage for a short while or for a long time. The cook may boil several different types of cabbage and may cover the boiled cabbage in a tasty sauce or a knob of butter impregnated with aromatic herbs. Delicious! But no fruit cake will be produced and enjoyed at the birthday party. No amount of elegant debate could alter this fact. Even by putting a new spin on the facts, unfortunately, the truth will remain unaltered. The bottom line will be that there may be plenty of delicious cabbage but there will be no fruit cake at the birthday party.

How would your client be encouraged to self-heal?

Will your client summon the help that she might need from within herself? Your client may, with luck, possess some form of inner magic or spiritual wisdom on which you can capitalize in an inventive way when treating her. You should, in most cases, be able to find some means of activating your client's innate self-correcting wisdom in a creative manner.

Will your client possess her own healing magic?

If you can somehow tap into your client's particular set of personal healing resources, you may, then, be able to make her path that little bit more tolerable. Some judicial enquiry on your part may allow you to identify your client's beliefs about the way in which she could take a positive and an active part in assisting her own recovery process. You might, also, endeavor to invent a clever device that will encourage your client to experiment with imaginative strategies for her self-healing mission and, if necessary, to suspend any disbelief in the interests of her own progress. If your client can be imbued with a sound belief in herself and her own powers of recovery, your job will usually be made infinitely much easier. After all, if your client's imaginative powers can be invoked and developed, this may be a useful exercise, in itself, that will stand her in good stead for her future existence long after she has left your consulting room.

Your client's own inner mind may be susceptible to symbolic imagery that could sustain her in times of crisis. Progress and comfort can often be attained by your client if she can be encouraged to see herself, for instance, as the nurturing mother, the ministering angel, the fearless tiger or the superhero. If your client proves to be a staunch believer in metaphysical law, for instance, you can often invite her to invoke healing entities, such as spirit-guides, guardian-angels, totem-animals, devas and etheric messengers. You might, also, invite your client to summon some natural healing resources, such as planetary energies, universal wisdom and the healing powers of the seasons.

Your client may, of course, be merely content with some meditative practice or some simple creative visualization in order to sustain her along the way. Your client's repertoire of creative healing strategies may be restricted only by the limitations of her own imagination. Your client, on the other hand, may not need any such devices, other than a little reassurance from you, if she simply possesses single-minded determination and wholehearted focus.

Ask yourself . . .

Does your client realize that she has an inner advisor who holds all the wisdom that she will ever need for recovery? Does your client appreciate that symbolic or archetypal imagery can be employed to good effect? Does your client have enough imagination in order to initiate her own healing processes? Can your client regularly utilize meditative practice or creative visualization for her own benefit? Can your client call on her guardian-angel in order to assist her in times of crisis? Could your client relate to the powers of the earth, the sea and the skies? Can your client appreciate the universe in all its majesty as her personal healing facility? Does your client reign supreme in the heavens or on the earth? Can your client draw on planetary energies or on universal guidance in order to assist herself? Has your client yet met her spirit power-animal and activated her self-healing mechanism in this way? Does your client have a good support-network in times of distress? Does your client have the backing of her friends and her family in order to support her on her healing mission? Does your client simply need the sheer determination to succeed and nothing more?

Let's take an example – Benedict's story

Benedict works as a spiritual psychotherapist who employs past-life regression with some of his clients. Benedict's client had been involved in a serious road accident in which he was run over as a pedestrian. Benedict's client had received emergency surgery in order to save his life but, unfortunately, both his legs had, of necessity, been amputated. Following this life-crippling experience, Benedict's client had, then, plunged into a deep state of depression and was very seriously considering suicide because his existence had, now, become intolerable and he felt that he had no prospect for future happiness.

Benedict decided to assist his client with past-life regression therapy to which he readily agreed. Once Benedict's client had been regressed, he found himself in a past life as a centurion in ancient Rome. Benedict's client, then, recounted an episode, in this former life, in which he had killed one of his slaves by mercilessly running over his legs with his chariot. Benedict's client, then, realized, to his horror, that the face of this dead slave was the same as the face of the man who had run him over and caused such devastation in his current life. As a consequence of this vivid and painful recollection, Benedict's client, thus, found a way of accepting that his current-life trauma was directly a karmic influence and a karmic form of justice. Benedict's client was, by this means, able to come to terms with his depressive state and his disabling physical condition.

Let's take an example – Voltimand's story

Voltimand practices spiritual healing and began to specialize in treating terminal cases. Voltimand's client had heard of his reputation and had approached him because she was suffering from severe polymyalgia that had reduced her to being virtually immobilized with exhaustion and extremely depressed as a result of her critical condition. Voltimand's client was elderly and on high doses of steroids that were supposed to be keeping her alive but she was given no hope of recovery by her medical practitioners. At her first session, Voltimand's client stated, most em-

phatically, that she did not believe in spiritual healing but that she was desperate enough to try anything because of her dismal prognosis.

Voltimand treated his client with his healing techniques for several months as well as providing her with some creative visualization assignments that she could undertake between her sessions. During this period of treatment, Voltimand slowly watched his client begin to lead a more normal life. Voltimand's client soon started not only to lift her depression but also to become more mobile. Perhaps more importantly, Voltimand's client was able to reduce her intake of steroidal drugs to a low dosage and she continued to progress as a result. In this case, Voltimand's client was given the hope that she needed of being able to lead a reasonably normal existence, despite her condition, and she was able to go from strength to strength, without ever knowing how or why her healing had worked so successfully.

Will you possess your own healing magic?

When considering healing resources, you should, of course, consider your own mechanism for assisting yourself as well as helping your client. If you have already established your healing powers and similar helpful devices, then, all will be well. You could, however, extend your repertoire of healing abilities by investigating the entire range of systems on which you could draw.

At a fundamental level, of course, you will need to possess a sound self-belief in your personal ability as a therapeutic agent for your client. This self-trust will usually be obtained more easily by self-investigative methods and will frequently manifest naturally once you have completed your initial training course and have successfully set up in practice. Remember that your own unique healing journey will be your fundamental passport to becoming an effective therapeutic practitioner.

If you work within the metaphysical realm, then, contacting your healing helpers will, almost certainly, be an integral part of your initiation into the profession. If your work would not normally embrace any invocation of healing assistance, then, perhaps, you could meditate in order to find a healing assistant, such as a wise counsel, a spirit-guide or a totem-animal, who could assist you in your daily work. Often this exercise of creative visualization will, in itself, be enormously beneficial both for you and for your client, regardless of whether or not you believe in metaphysical philosophy.

Ask yourself . . .

Do you have a strong belief in yourself and your own personal wisdom? Do you just know deep down that you can help your client by healing her and enriching her life? Can you suspend disbelief in yourself and strive for inner wisdom? Can you discover or develop your own special healing powers through meditation or creative visualization? Do you have a metaphysical connection with healing energies? Have you yet contacted your own healing spirit-guides? Have you met and made a connection with your spirit power-animals? Can you regularly call on your personal helpers in order to enhance your therapeutic work? Can you accept that you are a healing vehicle through which to channel your client's pain? Do you have someone to whom you can turn when things get tough for you as a therapeutic practitioner? Will your practice supervisor be someone who acknowledges the importance of your personal therapeutic powers? Can you keep in regular contact with fellow-practitioners who may be able to help you over any major hurdles? Can you simply have faith in yourself without the need for any external assistance? If you lack self-belief, can you work with another practitioner in order to obtain it for yourself? Can you find an effective way of strengthening and enhancing your self-confidence?

Let's take an example – Hecate's story

Hecate works as a metamorphic technique therapist. As Hecate developed her work and built up her practice, she found herself challenged by some interesting cases. With success, moreover, Hecate herself began to suffer from the rigors of running a successful practice and over-work started to seep into her life. At this juncture, Hecate decided to take some time out in order to attempt to self-heal.

While surfing the internet one day, Hecate became fascinated by the concept of healing spirits and decided to explore the idea of using totem-animals as employed in shamanic healing practice in order to assist her with her vocation. Previously, Hecate had, notionally, called on the powers of the universe in order to provide general advice and the expansion her practice and, so, this latest interest was merely an extension of that mode of working.

Hecate, consequently, decided to meditate on the theme of acquiring a spirit power-animal and, during a rest period, she undertook this task. Within about 24 hours, Hecate found herself living virtually permanently with a black panther totem-animal who began to assist her in numerous ways. This animal instantly became her trusted friend, her companion, her guide, her helper in times of difficulty and her own personal healing-agent. Hecate found herself more connected with this creature than any other form of healing device that she might have employed in the past. With this new-found friend, Hecate, thus, became personally empowered in her profession and gained even more success and job-satisfaction than she had previously when treating her client.

Would your client fully understand the healing crisis concept?

Will your client really be destined to stay the course when the ride might start to get bumpy? Your client will need to understand and be willing to undergo any healing crises that may ensue as a necessary part of her healing journey. The extent to which your client may be able to fully appreciate this phenomenon, and, accordingly, to put in the appropriate effort in order to weather the storm, may be the deciding factor in terms of her therapeutic success.

Will your client grasp the significance of her healing crisis?

Essentially, your client will be required to divorce herself from the impression that her symptoms will be treated by you and that she can simply sit back and enjoy the trip. Your client, in these circumstances, may not actually appreciate that undergoing alternative therapy could run the whole gamut of emotional distress, physical discomfort and painful experience for her when necessary.

If your client becomes disconsolate at the prospect of her adverse healing reactions, perhaps, you can serve to reassure her that this predicament will only be her natural survival instinct being activated in order to provoke her self-healing and to restore her healthy balance. Moreover, this process of your client's healing evolution will have begun long before she ever set foot in your consulting room. You may need to remind your client that her symptoms themselves, in whatever form, are, in essence, a healing crisis that has arisen organically from her own intelligent system. Empower your client to cling on to the fact that her healing crisis will, in some way, be revisiting and, hence, will be clearing an aspect of her past distress or her ill-health and that this will inevitably be unpleasant for her while she might be transitting this phase. Keep firmly in mind the notion that when your client contacts any past experience, then, this revisitation, in itself, will be a clear indication that her self-healing mechanism may be gearing up to resolve her problem permanently. On the positive side, of course, your client should benefit from that awe-inspiring feeling of wellbeing and optimism that will accompany her inner recognition of the road to recovery. Once her healing aggravation has abated, your client can, then, reap the justifiable rewards of relief and self-satisfaction.

Your client should, also, attempt to detach herself from the outcome of her therapeutic journey in order to avoid any self-blame when her progress might appear to be painfully slow. The weight-watcher or the body-builder will gain nothing by constantly jumping on the bathroom scales. Once your client has relinquished the habit of judging by results, she will, then, be allowing her natural wisdom to do its necessary work in its own time and, by this means, the end result will often be more than pleasing for her. Even when your client might appear to be fully prepared for and willing to undergo the pain-for-gain procedure, of course, she may still find it a million times harder than she originally expected. Stepping out of her comfort-zone can be quite a daunting prospect and an unpleasant ordeal for even your most resilient client.

Occasionally, you will find that your client will not fit into the ideal category of being prepared to pay the necessary price for recovery and your decision will, then, be focused on whether you will still want to work with her. Remember that you do have choice here and, so, you can, if you wish, politely but firmly decline to see any client with whom you do not desire to work for any reason whatsoever. Obtaining job-satisfaction should be uppermost in your mind when such a decision needs to be taken by you because this frame of mind will benefit your client enormously.

Ask yourself . . .

Will your client be able to appreciate, at a very deep level, that her presenting symptoms are merely effects and not necessarily the cause of her disorder? Can your client grasp the notion that her symptoms themselves are, in fact, a part of her healing phenomenon? Will your next client be the exception to all the rules and be the perfect specimen in terms of weathering her healing crisis? Will your client set out on the road to recovery with the appropriate equipment? Do you believe that your client will be adequately prepared for the journey ahead? Will your client's therapeutic voyage and her healing process be straightforward and uneventful? Can your client focus on traveling rather than on arriving? Could your client let go of monitoring her symptoms and of expecting them to resolve overnight? Does your client regard her therapeutic journey as a casual part-time activity designed to pamper her or to relieve her boredom? Can you persuade your client to view any unpleasant healing aggravations as a passport to her success? Does your client have the ability to contact her own inner wisdom that can transport her through any difficult phases of her recovery program?

Will you really be able to handle your client's healing crisis?

In helping your client to work through the many healing crises that she may need to face, you should, of course, ensure that you will play your part adequately. Your initial role might be to warn your client of any likely or any known repercussions of your therapy by way of any healing crises. You could prepare the ground in advance by explaining gently to your client that you are not a quick-fix, no-pain, comfort-zone merchant. Perhaps you can encourage your client to believe that traversing her healing crises can be a welcomed part of the process, however painful and discouraging this predicament may be to endure. Often your client can be pacified by a well-timed yet gentle pep-talk, a modicum of encouragement and much sincere praise for what she has achieved to date as your contribution to helping her to overcome this hurdle.

With any form of body-oriented therapy or medicinally-oriented practice, you may need to give encouragement to your client if she experiences pain and discomfort. You might even need to consider adjusting your treatment or your remedies accordingly so that your client can cope with anything untoward. With psychological therapies, the secret will always be for you to allow your client to fully discharge any emotional pain and any distress as a means of releasing her pent-up anguish that can do so much damage if it remains unexpressed. Quashing negative expression or painful experience can be an easy trap in which to fall especially when your client may be in visible distress before your very eyes. Your client's cathartic release, however, will be a vital passport for her therapeutic recovery.

In cases when your client may be required to undergo a reaction, or a process, that would be completely outside your domain, she may be advised to see another practitioner simultaneously. Because most healing will touch your client's emotional responses, for instance, you should be alert to the fact that she may need to be directed towards a mind-oriented practitioner if this might not be your field of expertise. Moreover, if you work in the psychological arena, your client may, also, need to consult a body-oriented or a medicinally-oriented practitioner in order to support the useful work that she has accomplished under your umbrella.

You should bear in mind, of course, that, at all times, regardless of your methodology, your client will be working at her own pace when undergoing any crisis reactions. Remember that your client will only manifest a healing crisis when the time is opportunely right for her and when she can cope with its severity. This will often be a sobering thought for you to hold on to when on the stormy seas with your client.

You may find that your client will appear to have what it takes to stay the course but, as soon as the going might appear to get harsh, she will, unfortunately, resort to self-sabotage and self-deception because these options might seem a more comfortable alternative to what you have to offer. Worst still, your client may veer towards blaming you when she starts to suffer or her symptoms are aggravated. Fret not if this situation does occur for your client because it will ultimately not be your responsibility. If in any doubt about your client's progress, you should seek help from your supervisor or advice from another practitioner. Do not flounder about in silence trying to solve an insoluble problem yourself when your client might currently be struggling or simply not getting there.

Ask yourself . . .

Have you taken time out to point out the significance of your client's healing reactions to her? Can you find a way of explaining the healing phenomenon in an understandable and in a palatable form to your client? Can you provide comfort and support during your client's most difficult periods? Can you encourage your client in such a way that she will not be afraid of or deterred from weathering the healing-crisis storm? Can you clearly identify your client's schemes for tackling her own problems? Do you fully understand what will be expected of your client during her therapeutic journey? Can you allow your client to tell it like it is and to express her feelings wholeheartedly about her condition? Do you feel that your client should, additionally, seek assistance from one of your colleagues in a related field in times of crisis? Do you consider that your client might be blaming you for the ups and downs of her own healing process? If your client holds you responsible for her healing suffering, who will she be able to blame for her original symptoms? Are you in need of any support yourself in order to help you to manage your client's healing process?

Let's look at it another way – Making hay while the sun shines

The farmer had waited patiently for many months for his crop to ripen and for several fine days so that he could reap his harvest and could take it to market. The farmer had judged that the corn would, now, be ripe for harvesting. The farmer had consulted the elements and, so, believed that the weather would be clement for the foreseeable future. The farmer, then, gathered his workers and informed them that there will be an early start tomorrow. The night before, all possible preparations are made for the forthcoming harvest and the prospect of a fruitful reap.

At break of day on the following morning, the farm-workers rise with the lark and prepare for a day of hard work but with high expectations. The tractor and the combine-harvester will come into their own and all hands will be on deck. From dawn to dusk the workers toil but the fruits of their labors hold promise and wealth beyond all dreams. Once the harvest has been reaped, the farm-cart can be loaded to the brim with produce that will fetch a pretty penny down at the market. The farm-workers will need to push the cart uphill, however, in order to get it to its destination but that extra effort will be well worth the lost perspiration. With one final push, the cart reaches the top of the hill and from there it can coast with ease all the way down to the market.

The farm's produce sells at record prices and the farm-workers are handsomely rewarded for their devoted efforts. The workers can, henceforth, look forward to more days of labor in order to reap additional rewards. The cart can be saluted for doing its work and all can retire to bed happy, wealthy, contented and optimistically looking forward to the future, despite suffering currently from extreme exhaustion. Can you make hay while the sun shines and fruitfully reap the harvest?

Let's take an example – Cordelia's story

Cordelia, a practitioner of acupuncture and traditional Chinese medicine, was a successful therapist who was able to help her clients to move mountains. Cordelia found, however, that the more successful she was at helping others, the more demanding her clients would become. Successful results, therefore, brought trouble in its wake for Cordelia.

One of Cordelia's clients, for instance, would ring up at unsociable hours, would expect to speak to Cordelia at the drop of a hat and would want to chat for ages. Cordelia's client might, furthermore, ring several times during a working day as well as sending her several emails in desperation. When contact was finally made, Cordelia's client would definitely not expect to have to wait any length of time for an appointment. With a busy schedule, however, Cordelia was not able to accommodate her demanding client and was running the risk herself of suffering from total exhaustion as a result of her own success. Cordelia's demanding client might have simply been undergoing a healing crisis but did not seem prepared to let it take its course without pressing the panic-button.

The solution was discovered when Cordelia consulted her supervisor who suggested that she create a telephone answering message that stated that she was only available to talk personally on the phone during certain hours of the day. This important information was, subsequently, conveyed by Cordelia, in no uncertain terms, to all her new clients. Cordelia, therefore, found the answer to her problem by explaining tactfully to her client where the boundary-lines reside. Any potentially-demanding client was, thus, forewarned as a means of preventing the panic that would have dire consequences for Cordelia later.

Would your client truly wish to recover?

Will your client have her own hidden agenda by any chance? You may earnestly desire to meet an endless stream of perfectly well-behaved clients from whom you can obtain exemplary results and colossal job-satisfaction. The unconscious healing impetus, however, can only emanate from within your client. Be aware that any underlying motivation that your client may secretly harbor about failure will, undoubtedly, rise to the surface, at some point, during her treatment. If your client has built an impenetrable wall around herself that will be indestructible, then, no amount of remedies, lotions, potions, pills, counseling, pleading or persuasion from you will ever shift this insurmountable obstacle to her success.

Will your client be wholeheartedly dedicated to recovery?

With luck your client will really want to improve her health and will be determined to succeed. In order to win the game, of course, your client will naturally need to take full responsibility for her own healing process and her health maintenance program. You may, however, only occasionally, meet your ideal client who will comply with all your instructions to the letter and will make stupendous progress as a result. Regrettably, in practice, the majority of your clients may be just the ordinary guy in the street.

As a physical therapist, you may vainly hope that your client will be prepared to really relax, be aware of her own body, be able to attune to its functioning, be able to cooperate fully with you and be committed to undertaking the appropriate forms of exercise in order to restore healthy functioning. Your client, moreover, may need to avoid physical exercise for a short period while her system readjusts even though somehow pressure of work, or that exciting all-night party, might prevent her from being sensible. At this point, resorting to painkillers or to discontinuing her treatment will not provide your client with any long-term relief from her current discomfort.

As a practitioner of biochemical medicine, you may, similarly, hunger for your client not to pollute her body with chemicals, drugs, cosmetic aids and junk-food. You may, of course, have to become resigned to the fact that your client will not be willing to perform a bowel cleanse or to undertake a lengthy fast. You may, also, feel despondent when your client persists in burning the candle at both ends and when she does not take her prescribed remedies or her supplements regularly.

As a practitioner of psychological therapy, you may long for your client to be prepared to access and to express her innermost emotions and to delve deeply into her psyche in order to resolve her problems at the root-cause level. You may, of course, find it an uphill struggle to convince your client that her healing will need to entail contacting and expressing her deepest emotions in order to bring about catharsis. Your client, for instance, may not wish to investigate the past and will confine herself to the belief that her troubles have manifested exclusively in the present.

As a spiritually-oriented healer, you may wish for your client to maintain a sound belief in spiritual evolution. You may, also, desire that your client be open to the process of energetic transformation and not put up any resistance to the upheaval of rebalancing her energy-centers. Your client, for instance, may wish to evade the responsibility of reviewing her life purpose and, consequently, of making those painful adjustments that may be needed in order to become spiritually fulfilled.

Ask yourself . . .

Might your client be an all-time total resistance merchant? Will your client take the remedies, do the visualizations and make a note of her dreams? Do you think that your client will perform her exercises, will change her diet, will take rest when required, will undertake any homework and will, generally, go with the flow? Have you yet identified your client's self-imposed obstacles to her successful recovery? Will your client realize that there may need to be pain before she can secure gain? Are you being realistic about your client's efforts to comply with your instructions? Are you becoming disheartened because your client might not be pulling her weight? Are you focusing on job-satisfaction to the exclusion of all else?

Will you be able to give your client a helping hand?

Your average client may truly desire success but, perhaps, understandably, she will want it now, want it without any pain and without disturbing the even tenor of her life, despite the fact that her existence might have become intolerable. This may be human nature or merely the road down which the so-called advanced and prosperous world has pushed your client.

A readiness to put in the work in order to achieve the goal can often only begin when your client decides to take off her blindfold and to behold her life realistically. When your client has removed the scales from her eyes, she may be able to appreciate that her symptoms are not the cause of her dilemma, that she alone can become her own savior and that the road to reaching her goal may be bumpy, hazardous, inconvenient and disagreeable.

Your role as a practitioner, in many cases, may largely be to cajole, to entice, to gently persuade or to earnestly encourage your reluctant client to screw her courage to the sticking-post. Your function can, unfortunately, only be in a supportive capacity because it will be your client who must do the work. It will be your client who must go with the flow in order to activate her self-healing mechanism and to rediscover her own mind, body and spirit at her own pace.

In all cases, you might be advised to learn to detach yourself from the outcome of your client's treatment. If you can be a dedicated professional, as well as being an interested observer, you will not take on too many of your client's concerns and anxieties over her personal recovery process. Leave the responsibility where it should be – with your client – and get on with your job of being a facilitator and not a mother-hen. Remember that you should merely be the catalyst for your client and not the activist. Furthermore, if you over-identify with your client's therapeutic outcome, you may be making a rod for your own back when she fails to make the grade. You may also, inadvertently, be putting unconscious pressure on your client to succeed by being over-interested in her therapeutic outcome and in her ability to achieve a harmonious lifestyle.

Ask yourself . . .

Are you gaining job-satisfaction from the majority of your clients or are you toiling away under the strain of trying to fit the proverbial square peg into the round hole? Are you finding life an uphill struggle with your client? Do you find yourself trying too hard with your client? Have you done all that you possibly can to advise your client accordingly and to support her through her healing crises? Can you allow your client to appreciate the way in which she has made progress as a result of her former healing crises? Can you stop blaming yourself for your client's lack of progress when you know perfectly well that her heart might not really be in it? Can you find a detached way of seeing your client through any reservations that she may have about her chances of recovery? Do you have any faith that your client will eventually see it like it is and get down to work? Do you feel as if you are bashing your head against an unswerving brick wall with your client? Can you fire your client up with the courage to face her healing crises when necessary? Can you completely detach yourself from your client's outcome as a means of paving the way for her to make progress? Are you insidiously pressurizing your client into being one of your greatest success stories?

Would your client wish to impede her own progress?

Will you have discovered your client's personal trip-up mechanisms yet? You could ponder on the fact that deep down your client may actually not wish to get better at all because she may not desire to face the consequences of her emergence from ill-health. Amazingly enough, your client may not, in essence, welcome the change that will inevitably come about in her life if she does, in fact, stay the entire course. When push comes to shrove, your client may not, in reality, be prepared to undergo the pain of letting go and the discomfort of bringing about the necessary change. Your client may, of course, have the correct ingredients but she may not know how to read the recipe's instructions on the packet.

Will you spot the fly in your client's ointment?

At some point during your client's therapeutic journey, she may want to get out of jail free. Your client may, indeed, appear to be the ideal candidate for your therapy but rest assured that she will, at some stage, flag in enthusiasm, in determination and in resolve. Your greatest hope, in these circumstances, can only be that your client will, somehow, find the wherewithal to pull herself through any coat-dragging blips on the horizon.

Keep a watching brief on signs of resistance or of defeatist thinking in your client. The clues may be many and varied with plenty of excuses to support your client's retrograde action. Your client may, for example, want to cancel her sessions, may arrive late, may forget to take her medication or will simply trot off to see her doctor in order to obtain the antidote to your therapeutic remedies. Your client will usually be full of ready-made excuses and protestations at such times. Your client may have become so accustomed to wearing a blindfold that she does not even realize that it sits on the end of her nose. Your client's actions and attitudes, therefore, will tell you all about the position from whence she comes.

Your client may, furthermore, possess a somewhat misguided notion of what might be helpful to her in terms of her recovery process. Your client may, for example, expect to rely on antidepressants, on sleeping draughts or on painkillers as the obvious cure for all her troubles. Your client may have little or no awareness of the fact that chemical drugs may seriously impede her progress by suppressing her healing crises and further detoxifying her system. Your client may often still be in quick-fix mode and may retain the mindset whereby she will consider that a pill will simply do the trick where you have failed. At the start of therapy, therefore, it might be advisable for you to explain the effects of taking any chemical medication that may significantly hamper your client's progress and could create a closed mind.

Your client may, of course, just be entrenched in a lifestyle that she would not desire to relinquish in a hurry. Your client, for example, may be utterly discontent with her life partner yet will not wish to forego her comfortable existence in order to start afresh or will be reluctant to disturb her children. A major heal-ing shift, in these circumstances, therefore, would definitely upset your client's cozy little apple-cart and she just might not want to rock that particular boat.

Your client may, also, choose a given therapy because she simply wishes to bide her time and not make much progress at all. The main watch-word, in this situation, will be for you not to chastise yourself for failure or to kill yourself trying to change your client's attitude. Getting on target will be your client's re-sponsibility, not yours, and staying stuck will be her funeral.

Ask yourself . . .

Does your client smile and reassure you that she really wants to go for it and yet you have little real evidence to support her claim? Will your client have given the matter of her own health some forethought or will she simply be drifting from raft to raft? Will your client be content to bash her head against the wall or does she earnestly believe in her own recov-ery capabilities? Would your client be willing to sacrifice all for the sake of improving her health? Would your client be willing to invest time, money, effort and inconvenience in the process of change and recovery? Would your client be over-burdening herself with emotional distress or with spiritual malaise and will this, consequently, mean that she will go around in circles and get nowhere fast? Does your client continue to smoke, to drink or to take drugs because she simply has no faith in the possibility of longevity? Does your client persist in utterly exhaustive over-work or in punishing physical exercise that will significantly impede her progress? Does your client permit some form of lifestyle toxicity that will be a dead-weight for her to carry around? Does your client expect you to provide the antidote to her diet of junk-food, recreational drugs or environmental pollutants? Would your client be entertaining a partner-ship and/or a friendship network neither of which will be, in any way, supportive of her recovery mission?

Let's look at it another way – Heading north

If you live in London and want to visit Edinburgh, it would be advis-able for you to travel in a northerly direction. It matters not what form of transport you select, or how long your journey will take, but you must ensure that your compass is pointing north before you set out. If you are per-

verse, for some extraordinary reason, and, so, decide to travel south, instead, you will not get to your intended destination.

You may, of course, arrive in some pleasant and wonderful place where the climate might be warm and the people are friendly. You may, by chance, actually like it there and, maybe, find it even better than being stuck in the bleak highlands. Perhaps you will settle down and make the most of it? Perhaps you will, now, be glad that you made an error when reading the map and will like the climate much more that chilly Scotland? Maybe there will have been compensations for your error of judgment and, so, why worry about such a mistake? Could it have all turned out for the best in the end?

You may, understandably, be a little confused in that these southern countrymen do not speak with a Scottish dialect and do not go around wearing kilts and playing bagpipes. Moreover, you may miss the oatcakes and the fresh salmon. You may, also, pine for the mountains, the glens and the brays of which you have heard so much. Your camping equipment or your skiing gear may not, now, be needed. Your swimwear and your sun-hat, of course, you have left behind.

But the fact remains that you did not get to Scotland because you went in the wrong direction completely. You will never know what it would have been like to have, in reality, carried out your plans and fulfilled your dream to visit Scotland's capital at that particular time in your life. Perhaps you can console yourself by saying that you will travel north next year? But what would it have been like at that chosen point in your life? You will never know and it may be that you may never actually get there in the future. Perhaps you made that error on purpose? Maybe you can never rectify it? How will you find your true destination?

Would your client expect you to be a miracle-worker?

If your client blames you for everything, what will be the next item on her agenda? If your client cannot become whole-heartedly committed to her own treatment-program, she may, in consequence, expect you to be a worker of miracles by one tiny wave of your magic wand.

Will your client blame you when she fails?

Your intransigent client will be the one who will expect more of you in the mistaken belief that her health must be your ultimate responsibility. Your uncommitted client may make a profession out of blaming you but you do not need to pick up the gauntlet.

If your client has a fundamental misconception about the function of alternative therapy, she may, conveniently, wish to believe that you must be a wizard. Your client's opinions may be openly stated or else more surreptitiously expressed by a minute facial gesture or an infinitesimal air of despair. If your client resorts to blaming an external agent, of course, she can often spare herself any unnecessary inconvenience and, simultaneously, give herself the impression that she has done all in her power by passing the buck on to you. Safe in this cocoon, your client can, essentially, avoid addressing her major issues, can blissfully indulge in self-deception and can use you as the nearest whipping-post in order to ensure that her resistance to change will remain intact.

Do not be fooled by your client's evasive tactics or her buck-passing ploys. Do not allow your own psyche to be seduced into believing that your client's failures are a direct reflection of your competence. If your client wishes to get well, that will be just great. If your client wishes to remain in ill-health, in unhappiness and in self-deception, that can be fine also. Your role will simply be to be there when your client wants to go for the ride. You are only the vehicle but your client must agree to take the opportunity to buy the ticket and to make the journey.

You may need to repeatedly explain to your client the process of recovery in the alternative arena but do not become despondent when sometimes your protestations may fall continually on deaf ears. By all means encourage your client to succeed but do not make any exaggerated claims or feed her with any false hopes. Let your client make the choice from the impartial information that you have provided and leave the buck there. Healing work must come from your client and the results of her efforts will pay handsomely but she can only discover this doctrine for herself.

If your client might be showing signs of flagging and you are becoming disheartened, as a result, it will often be a good idea for you to compare the performance of your most successful client with that of your least successful client. By this means, you can start to get things into proper perspective and can learn to detect when your client might only be lukewarm about her self-healing journey. All your client can ever do in therapy will be to take the opportunities that you can present. You can do your bit by striking while the iron is hot but, of course, remember that you are always firing at a moving target with your client. Your client may appear compliant today, perchance, but she may become utterly unenthusiastic tomorrow. Sometimes your client will improve noticeably during a session and sometimes markedly between sessions. Occasionally, your client will show no detectable improvement at all over a relatively long period of time but that may be her unique way of operation and cannot be significantly altered by you by any direct intervention.

Ask yourself . . .

Do you desire to bring your magic wand into the consulting room? Does your client have ultimate failure written on her brow? Can your client accept that it will be her responsibility to get well and that the ultimate onus will not fall on you in any way? Can your client acknowledge that she needs to do most of the spadework herself? Does your client turn up for her appointments regularly, arrive ready to begin work and pay your fee gladly? Does your client complain politely that the remedies that you have given her were not really very effective? Will your client imply that her symptoms have not really improved much, despite attending your clinic for several sessions? Will your client mention casually that she had gained better results when applying the cream from the chemist or when taking the antibiotics? Are you disturbed by your client's complaints or her supposed criticisms of your work?

Let's take an example – Perdita's story

Perdita practices homeopathy and administers vibrational essences and had been in practice for a number of years. Perdita's client consulted her because of a serious skin disorder that was causing her a great deal of despair and embarrassment. Perdita prescribed remedies and essences for her client and instructed her that she would need to report any aggravations, any upheavals, any changes or any progress regularly by phone.

At her next session, Perdita's client complained that there had been absolutely no improvement in her condition. Perdita noted that her client had not kept in contact between sessions and had, also, neglected to take her prescribed medication as instructed. Perdita's client, however, got a bit obstreperous when this fact was gently pointed out to her. Perdita, then, became insistent that her client needed to follow her instructions, to take the prescribed remedies and to make regular contact by phone so that her progress could be monitored.

After the session, however, Perdita began to feel bad about the situation with her client and to indulge in self-blame. Perdita tended to take her work far too seriously and, then, to feel despondent if her client showed signs of dissatisfaction or evidence of lack of improvement. On later reflection, however, Perdita began to examine the facts of her client's case. Perdita considered that her client had not been pulling her weight and, moreover, was attempting to blame her practitioner for her own lack of commitment. Keeping these facts squarely in mind, Perdita was, then, able to work through her own self-blaming tendencies and to see her client more realistically. Perdita, therefore, decided that she would be tougher with her client in future and that she would make a point of emphasizing the need for full cooperation. By this means, Perdita's client was forced to see it like it is and to take up the cudgels if she wished to resolve her condition.

How would you learn to empathize with your client?

Could you get into your client's mind and see what it might really be like in there? Imagination may be your most valuable asset when working with your client. Your fertile imagination will help you to understand your client's condition, to appreciate things from her point of view and to allow you to realize from whence she comes.

How will you imagine your client's state of being?

On many occasions, you will truly be able to empathize with your client because you will have already been there yourself. Your client, for instance, may be suffering from a condition that you have personally overcome. Your firsthand experience will, consequently, make the handling of your client's case much simpler because you can truly appreciate where she will be coming from and what she may need to experience along her healing road.

Your client whose presenting malaise does not fall within your compass of personal experience may, however, disconcert you. This situation will normally afford you the opportunity to employ your imagination and your intuition to the full. It should usually be possible for you to empathize, in some way, with your client by simply visualizing what it could be like to feel the physical pain, the emotional distress and the accompanying despondency. You could, also, purely imagine intuitively what your client may be thinking about her ill-health or about her debilitating condition. Moreover, it may be worth considering what you think your client feels about your therapeutic approach.

Your gift of creative visualization may be a form of intuitive healing that you could find very valuable in handling any out-of-the-ordinary cases. A relaxed state of mind can allow you to kinesthetically feel your client's condition yet remain suitably detached. Such practices may help you to come to terms with any unfamiliar case and will often have a beneficial outcome both for you and for your client. Your creative imagination should allow you to take a detached view of your client's case and not to get over-involved in trying to work out problems from a logical standpoint.

Ask yourself . . .

Can you imagine the kind of experience your client will be going through when she has suffered greatly for many years? Can you appreciate why your client has fallen victim to her disorder? Can you imagine your client's condition, her reaction to it and her outlook for her prospects of recovery? Can you picture the way in which your client might be feeling unwell most of the time? Can you imagine what it would have been like for your client lying on an operating table or bedridden from a long-term illness? Can you envisage what your client's reaction might have been when given the news that she has a serious, life-threatening condition? Can you imagine the effect of a traumatic childbirth experience that your client has previously endured? Can you estimate the way in which your client will view the prospect of her impending therapeutic journey? Can you view your client realistically by tuning into her frame of mind but not become bogged down by the minute details? Have you ever tried intuitive healing and can you appreciate the way in which these skills can easily be developing within you? Can you appreciate that you might unconsciously be attracting clients who will reflect your own health issues? Can you remain detached and objective when using your visualization skills?

How will you visualize your client's therapeutic journey?

Sometimes a visualization exercise will help you to understand what your client may be experiencing and the way in which she may be reacting to her therapeutic journey. You may find it useful to outline your client's healing process in terms of the way that she feels, the way that she copes with her healing crises and her attitude towards recovery. Intuitive visualization of your client's healing path will help you to empathize with her. Making an attempt to understand your client by this means will give you confidence and will bridge the gap between your personal experience and any knowledge that falls outside your familiarity-zone.

A creative visualization technique should not, of course, be an excuse for you to over-sympathize with your client. Do not, therefore, spend many hours in meditation over your client's condition but simply use a brief visualization technique when needed. Do not get so far into visualization practice that you become obsessed with your client's therapeutic resolution and your part in her recovery. Do not over-indulge in fantasy-land and end up vicariously traumatizing yourself by what your imagination might have dredged up for you about your client.

If your imagination, or your intuition, fails to assist you when empathizing with your client, then, question a fellow-practitioner who may have experience with a particular presenting disorder or a given set of symptoms. If your mind's eye lets you down, however, then, do not waste precious hours trying to find its monocle. Remember that imaginative, intuitive and creative visualization can only be borne out of your own past experience with a bit of tone-color sprinkled into the mixture for decoration.

Ask yourself . . .

Can you intuitively imagine what your client's healing crises may be like to endure? Can you imagine the ways in which your client could pull herself along her own healing path? Can you consider what your client's attitude to her recovery route might essentially be? Can you reflect on the way in which your client will be engaged in her own healing process? Can you imagine what it would be like if your client were trapped in a loveless or a violent intimate partnership? Can you picture what it might be like if your client were in financial difficulties or were destitute in any way? Can you consider what your client would be going through if she had been raped, been mugged or been the victim of abuse? Can you envisage what life might be like for your client if she were injured in a car crash or had broken a limb? Can you imagine what your client would feel like if she were suffering from anxiety attacks or from depression? Can you imagine what excruciating agony could feel like for your client? Can you consider your client's frame of mind at the time when she took drugs or when she led a wildly-stressful life? Can you see your client as a loser, a pessimist or a loner? Can you find a way of resonating with your client in order to feel the extent of her pain?

Let's take an example – Goneril's story

Goneril practices color healing and crystal healing and these practices have assisted her personally when she was overcoming a long-term, chronic-fatigue syndrome. Shortly after she began in practice, Goneril met a client who had just been diagnosed with breast cancer. Goneril's client was, of course, quite naturally, beset with indecision and anxiety about her condition and this factor obviously added to her dilemma.

At this point in Goneril's career, she had no experience of working with such a condition and she knew very little about cancer as a disease phenomenon. Goneril tackled her self-doubt problem by consulting several of her colleagues and some of her former tutors and, also, sought advice from various information sources. Ultimately, Goneril realized that, in order to understand her client's case, she would need to thoroughly acquaint herself with the facts about the disease and the treatment methods that were currently available. Moreover, Goneril appreciated that she would be required to stand back in order to attempt to see things exclusively from her client's viewpoint.

Goneril decided to use her creative imagination in the light of her new-found knowledge and she elected to simply allow her mind to do its work. Goneril discovered that, in fact, the most important aspect in the equation was her client's personal reaction to her condition. Goneril was soon able to intuitively grasp the way in which her client felt, how she was reacting and how she was changing her opinions about her condition as time progressed.

Goneril, thus, discovered her own intuitive ability to tune into her client and this facility took the heat out of her personal response to this new situation. With time, Goneril realized that her client was able to relinquish her anxieties and could make informed decisions about her future and her treatment route. From this point onward, Goneril began to relax and to focus on treating her client as impartially as she would any other. This daunting experience allowed Goneril to learn about herself and her healing abilities and she was, now, set to be able to successfully handle any client with a similar disorder in the future.

5 WHAT WOULD YOUR CLIENT BE TELLING YOU?

How would you understand your client accurately?

Will you be able to listen to your client at the front door yet hear her at the back door? There may often be a world of difference between what your client says openly and consciously in words and what she actually means subtly and unconsciously. Being alert to the true meaning of your client's messages will be one of your prime assets when treating her.

Will you ask your client the right questions?

As a therapeutic practitioner, your job will certainly involve asking your client some questions about herself and encouraging her to open up. This task, however, may become a more difficult uphill climb than you might first imagine. During any note-taking stage, when examining your client's case history, you will need to listen carefully to what she might be saying to you beneath the surface of her actual words. Apart from encouraging your client to speak freely, you may, also, be able to understand her by appreciating what she overtly says on the surface of the water and, yet, surreptitiously decipher her true meaning in the hidden depths.

Frequently your client will edit her own script in order to suit her purpose. Your client, for instance, may tell you what she wishes you to hear or simply say what she thinks you will want to know. Your client may even be patently unaware of what she needs to impart. In these circumstances, you will need to be a superlative super-sleuth in order to tease out of your client the inferences and the nuances of what she may be attempting to convey. In many instances, it may be that what your client does not tell you will, in fact, be of vital importance, despite the fact that she may be totally unaware of any gems that she might be concealing.

Potential sticking-points for your client may be numerous and frequent. Your intention may be for your client to say whether she feels happy with a live-in partner or to admit that she lives in constant pain from a backache. You may wish to review your client's stress-factor at work. You may want to encourage your client to confess that she has not rigidly stuck to her diet or to state whether or not she has regularly taken her prescribed remedies. You may need to know the way in which your client has allotted herself sufficient leisure-time. You might want to enquire whether your client has undertaken any homework that you might have set and how successfully, or otherwise, she might have accomplished these tasks. But normally your client will not want admit to any of her perceived misdemeanors or, perhaps, any complaints that she might have about her condition.

Ask yourself . . .

When you invite your client to speak about herself, what will be her true response? Will your client tell you the truth when she answers your questions? Will your client volunteer information or will she need to have the answers dragged out of her under protest? Does your client say what she thinks that you will want to hear because she might be trying to please you or because she might be attempting to deceive you minutely? Will your client be attempting to rebel against you because she sees you as an authority-figure or as a nosey-parker? Will your client be ashamed of the fact that she is unwell and that she might be causing you trouble as a result? Does your client not wish to admit that her life is in a mess? Will your client be likely to lag behind and, then, try to cover her tracks?

Does your client endeavor to confess all in the hope that you will not ask her any more questions in future? Does your client attempt to be intellectual in the hope that she can avoid exploring the emotional impact of her revelations?

Will you draw the right conclusions about your client?

Continual probing with your client in order to discover the nature of her health condition may be your key to ultimate success. You may, of course, need to frame your questions very carefully, or to pose them in several different ways, in order to allow your client's true picture to emerge. Your aim in questioning your client will be to elicit the precise facts of her case and to gauge any progress that she might already have made on her journey. From this vantage point, you can, then, make some form of assessment of your client and, if appropriate, arrive at some useful conclusion. Your interpretation of the facts that you have gathered can, then, often lead you to an understanding about the likely root cause of your client's dilemma and this, in turn, will give you the basis for action (see Figure 5.1 – *How might you formulate a therapeutic action plan for your client?*).

Once an action plan for your client's treatment-strategy has been formulated, you can, then, watch the flower growing and can accurately evaluate her progress and, if necessary, you can, then, adjust your methodology accordingly. Occasionally, your best course of action will be to bide your time in order to allow your client to unfold her story in her own way and at her own pace. In many instances, you may need to be fairly interventionist in the initial stages of therapy but later you may be able to take a definitive backseat while your client takes center stage and her system gets on with its imperative healing job. In most cases, your treatment and your handling of your client will follow a natural progression from initial information-gathering and reflection to instituting some form of closely-monitored strategy in order to render therapeutic assistance.

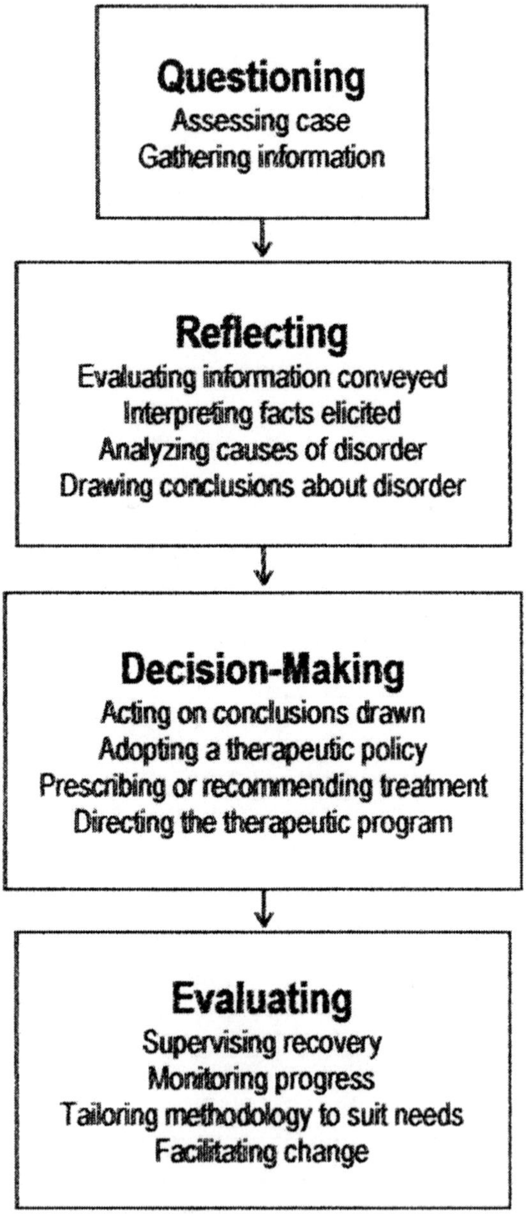

Questioning
Assessing case
Gathering information

Reflecting
Evaluating information conveyed
Interpreting facts elicited
Analyzing causes of disorder
Drawing conclusions about disorder

Decision-Making
Acting on conclusions drawn
Adopting a therapeutic policy
Prescribing or recommending treatment
Directing the therapeutic program

Evaluating
Supervising recovery
Monitoring progress
Tailoring methodology to suit needs
Facilitating change

Figure 5.1 – *How might you formulate a therapeutic action plan for your client?*

Ask yourself . . .

Can you take a backroad route in order to tease vital information out of your client? Do you need to pose your questions in another way in order to discover your client's personal truth? Does your client play down her distress and might she be frightened to admit, even to herself, the extent of her troubles? Would your client be too frightened to reveal all because she fears what you might think of her? Does your client feel that her case is not really serious because she considers it to be the norm? Would your client normally be of a timid and a retiring nature? Will your client really think that she should not make too much fuss because you are very busy with more deserving cases? Can you learn to generalize when you ask your client questions instead of putting words into her mouth? Can you acquire the art of reading between the lines and hear the truth beneath your client's words? Can you keep your views and your opinions out of the equation when listening to your client? Will your client be readily forthcoming about her condition or will she expect you to know all the answers? Can you formulate a treatment-strategy or an action-plan in order to facilitate your client's recovery program? Will your treatment need to be fairly interventionist or can you simply allow your client's healing journey to unfold?

Let's take an example – Lucetta's story

Lucetta, a reflexologist, began working with her client by asking him about his health picture, his psychological profile and his general background. Lucetta observed that her client was reasonably forthcoming in his replies to her questions but she was disturbed to discover that he had a serious death-wish and was quite open about the fact that he would prefer to be dead. Lucetta's client was a workaholic, a high achiever and an intellectualizer who stated openly that he did not wish to alter his stressful lifestyle. Lucetta, also, noted that her client was taking an almost lethal cocktail of nutritional supplements and pharmacological medication with this death-wish in mind.

Lucetta was indecisive about taking on her new client after her initial enquiry session but, following a discussion about this dilemma with a colleague, she decided to treat him for a limited time-span in the hope of allowing him to make a shift in his thinking during that period. Once treatment had begun, Lucetta became aware that her client did not have the support of his family and that, possibly, his wife could, in addition, do with some of her treatment. Lucetta, also, had an intuitive notion that her client might have suffered from some form of stress-inducing incident within the last 10 years that would have resulted in his seeking therapy. Lucetta, therefore, continued with her client giving him reflexology and some counseling and felt sure that, sooner or later, he would find the key to unlocking his own padlock but, however, the ultimate outcome could not be predicted.

Would your client be truly honest with herself?

Your client may know her truth but will she realize it herself or will she even wish to admit it to you? When you listen to your client, the first thing you will need to decipher may be whether she will be giving you an accurate answer to your questions and, thus, providing you with a precise account of the true facts.

Will your client know her personal truth?

Often your client may not be capable of telling it like it is. Your client may not be deliberately giving you a lot of hogwash and her motives may be entirely genuine but she simply may not yet know how to react in a therapeutic context. As an astute detective, nevertheless, you can usually learn to read between your client's surreptitious lines. Your first tactic may be to gain your client's confidence in order to overcome this knotty little obstacle to her progress. It will be important for you to remember that ultimately your client will need to be able to trust you but that the impetus for this conviction must come from her alone. You can, of course, pave the way and set the scene but, in some way, your client will need to overcome her natural reservations that, perhaps, may have emanated from an inability to trust others who have previously betrayed her.

When you ask your client a question, she may answer you in any one of four different ways depending on whether she can be truthful and be honest with herself. For instance, your client may say "yes" and really mean "yes" and, thus, give you a truthful answer. Your client may say "yes" but really mean "no" and, so, give you a deceptive reply. Your client may say "no" and really mean "no" and, hence, render an honest reaction to your question. Your client may say "no" but really mean "yes" and, therefore, provide you with a misleading response. The trick will be for you to decide which of these responses are actually what your client means to convey consciously or otherwise.

Let's look at it another way – Would you like a strawberry ice cream?

If your gracious party host asks you the question, "Would you like a strawberry ice cream covered in champagne sauce and topped with chopped nuts?", you may give several possible answers to this enquiry. You may say "yes" because you genuinely like ice cream, strawberries, champagne and nuts. Yum, yum! You may, also, be hungry, at the moment, and be craving some sweet food. This treat may really be your idea of heaven on earth and you will savor every mouthful. You said "yes" and you really meant "yes".

You may say "yes" but, then, instantly regret it and wish that your party host had not even asked you the question in the first place. You have been on a diet for several weeks and you do not, now, want to hinder the good progress that you have made in losing weight. You may, also, know from bitter experience that you will get a hangover from the champagne tomorrow morning. You realize that your host has spent many hours with loving care making this mouth-watering dessert and you feel that you do not wish to offend her. You may consider that you have already eaten enough and do not really want to eat anything else but are irresistibly tempted by the offer. Finally, you succumb and consume the entire dessert with an "Oh, what the heck?" philosophy. You may, alternatively, toy with the ice cream and feel guilty with every mouthful. You said "yes" but you really meant "no".

You may say "no" because you do not, by any means, have a sweet tooth. You may be the kind of person who would not eat ice cream at any price. You may be a non-drinker and, also, be allergic to nuts and, therefore, would avoid such a dessert like the plague. You may be so health-conscious that sweets and dairy produce are a definitive contravention of your entire philosophy on life. You said "no" and you really meant "no".

You may, of course, say "no" and, then, spend the rest of the evening regretting it. You may watch with envy as everyone else in the room indulges in this sumptuous dessert. You look about to see if there are any leftovers and even pinch a spoonful or two from someone else. You vainly hope that your host will ask you yet again just in case you have changed your mind but she does not and, so, you feel thoroughly miserable and dejected as a result. You said "no" but you really meant "yes". How would you have answered this brain-teasing question?

Let's take an example – Emilia's story

Emilia, a craniosacral therapist, asked her client about her childhood in her introductory session as part of her normal set of enquiries into her background. Emilia's client stated innocently that she had a normal and a happy childhood. Emilia's client claimed that no harm had befallen her in her life and yet, somewhat mysteriously, she found it difficult even to leave her house let alone engage in social activities with others.

During the course of her therapy, however, it transpired that Emilia's client had regularly been beaten by her father when she was a child. Emilia's client, however, genuinely felt that she was telling the truth when she had said that her childhood was normal and happy. Emilia's client, quite simply, felt that things had been normal because she knew no different. Emilia's client had assumed that she had obviously had a harmonious and undisturbed childhood because she had been fed, clothed, sent to school and had received enough money to spend. Emilia's client did not have the experience of life in order to appreciate that her upbringing had been harsh and abnormal and that she had, in effect, been physically and emotionally traumatized. Moreover, Emilia's client was still firmly entrenched in the belief that everything her parents had done must have been right, as if feelings of guilt and loyalty had overridden her mental capacity. Emilia's client could, therefore, not, in any way, relate her symptoms to what was likely to have constituted the originating cause of her distressful disorder.

Therapeutic intervention, in this case, served as the means to bridge the gap between what Emilia's client believed at the beginning of therapy and what she later learned to be her personal truth. Emilia, fortunately, was not fooled by her client's protestations of childhood wellbeing but simply persevered with her therapy and gave neither comment nor judgment on the situation. Emilia's client, therefore, gradually came to terms with her own truth in her own way and in the fullness of time and, as a result, her social life started to blossom.

Let's take an example – Borachio's story

Borachio works in the psychotherapeutic field and has built up an impressive toolkit of techniques that he employs with skill to the full. Borachio's extensive experience, however, has taught him to be keenly aware of what his client does not tell him. Borachio's client had suffered greatly from being dumped casually by her one true love in her youth and she was, generally, unable to accept compliments or to interact successfully with others. Borachio's client, also, reported much indecision about the choices that she currently had to make about her future and her relationship with her husband. Borachio's client was, for instance, indecisive about the possibility of emigrating.

After several sessions, it transpired that Borachio's client had experienced a poor relationship with her mother who was inconsolable when her own father had died. Borachio's client soon realized that her issues of being rejected and of shunning the affection of others was, consequently, a direct result of this early traumatic experience. Once Borachio's client had made these important realizations, she found herself on a noticeable upward trend and, virtually simultaneously, her mother had made contact and wanted to heal the rift. The channels of communication were, now, opened and both mother and daughter worked on building a viable future relationship. It was, also, an interesting coincidence that precisely when Borachio's client was ready to entertain her mother, following her therapeutic discoveries, this, synchronistically, was the moment at which her mother chose to get in touch. As a result of working with his client, Borachio became fascinated by the fact that she could and she would create her own reality-world.

At a subsequent session, Borachio's client reported that she had become pregnant and that, previously, she had been very indecisive about starting a family. Moreover, Borachio's client confessed that her personal indecision had put a strain on her marriage and had, formerly, rendered her unable to conceive. Borachio had been interested to note that this major issue for his client had not even been highlighted by her, at all, in the initial stages of her therapy. Borachio soon began to realize that his client would eventually reveal all in the fullness of time in order to accelerate her own healing process.

What would be your client's chances of ultimate success?

Will you be able to stand back in order to view your client from behind the glass? In assessing the overall picture of your client's chances of pulling herself through, you may need to holistically consider her health picture from a number of different angles. You may, for instance, wish to evaluate the effect of any external influences that may be pulling your client in the opposite direction. You might, furthermore, benefit from considering the kind of probing that you may be required to undertake with your client in order to establish her chances of restoring optimal health from her current position (see Figure 5.2 – *What might be your client's chances of success?*).

How will you understand your client's physiological profile?

You may wish to enquire about the extent of physiological damage or degenerative decay that your client may have sustained. Your principal line of questioning may focus on whether your client currently has robust health or whether she might be rapidly declining. A degenerative condition, for instance, may have been in evidence, symptomatically, for some time but, in reality, will have manifested even before your client had any conscious knowledge of her physical state.

If your client suffers from an incurable genetic weakness, it may be that your role will be simply to render her in a position whereby she can cope tolerably with her condition. An inherent diabetic condition or a major liver defect, for example, that your client may have sustained at conception, will be a hard fact that cannot be denied by her but she can, of course, do everything in her power to arrange her life around this not entirely insurmountable problem. A healthy diet, the appropriate nutritional supplementation, a sensible lifestyle and a stress-free existence will go a long way towards prolonging your client's life and towards keeping any potential disease or any health decline firmly at bay.

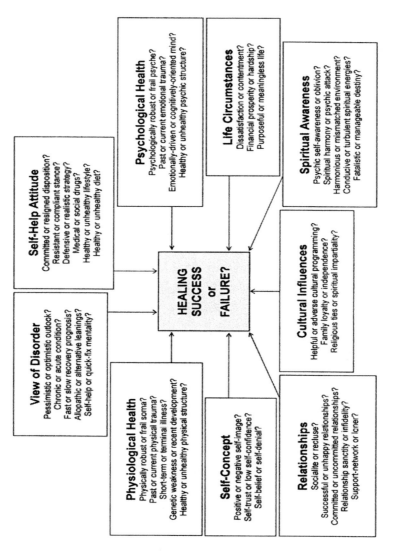

Figure 5.2 – *What might be your client's chances of success?*

You may, also, wish to evaluate your client's physicality and her somatic structure in terms of whether she might be making her condition worse by acting in an unwise manner. If your client persists in using an injured limb, for instance, she will not be giving it a full chance of recovery in the shortest possible timeframe. A poor body posture, furthermore, may exacerbate your client's physical disorder and may, also, depict her attitude of mind and her overall view of herself.

Ask yourself . . .

Does your client exhibit stamina and strength as the necessary resources in order to pull herself out of the quagmire? Will your client be suffering from a degenerative condition that will result in a battle against time? If your client has been suffering from a degenerative disorder, can you trace its routes back for many decades? Does your client exhibit a seemingly incurable condition when, in fact, this state has merely developed over time because of her ill-informed choices? What genetic weaknesses can you detect that will need to be handled carefully and responsibly by your client? Does your client have a genetic defect that will need to be constantly supported for the rest of her life? Is your client ever likely to be able to bring about a total cure for herself? Does your client believe that she has an incurable condition when, in fact, this could easily be remedied? Does your client's slouch convey an inability to hold herself erect or does this posture convey her pessimistic frame of mind?

How will you understand your client's psychological profile?

Whatever your therapeutic discipline, you will need to note your client's psychological state and any emotive reactions that could have a knock-on effect into other areas of her life. Often when your client enters any form of therapeutic consultation, she will need to address emotional issues that may stem from both the recent past and from her childhood distress. Bear in mind that in addressing your client's general health issues, there may well be an underlying psychological problem that could rear its ugly head, at any time, when you are administering treatment.

You may be able to tell much from your client's emotional nature and the detectable picture of her psychic health. It may be important for your client to be able to express her emotions in order to bring about her own recovery. For this reason, you may wish to consider whether your client will be primarily emotionally-driven or whether she will be cognitively-oriented. If your client can readily contact her emotional nature, she may be slightly better equipped to penetrate the depths of her soul and to reach the originating cause of her disorder. On the other hand, your client whose strength lies in cognitive prowess and intellectual abilities, at the expense of emotive expression, may not be so well placed.

Psychological help may sometimes be needed in addition to other forms of therapeutic intervention with your client. For your client whose emotive reactions are spiraling out of control, she will, undoubtedly, need some degree of psychologically-slanted assistance from a specialist quarter. If this might be your field of work, then, you can rub your hands with glee and get down to business with your client. If caring for your client's psychological health might not your forte, then, it would be wise for you to refer her to a known and trusted practitioner who specializes in this domain.

Ask yourself . . .

Will your client be able to express her emotions naturally and comfortably when necessary? Do your client's emotive responses flood out of her at the slightest provocation and might this be indicative of her sub-surface traumatic distress? Might your client's emotive expression be disturbing to you personally and making you feel out of your depth? Do you need to refer your client to another practitioner who would be better equipped to handle her emotive issues and her obvious psychological distress? Could your client be beset by a tendency to analyze everything too earnestly? Will your client be unable to appreciate her emotional nature because she might be hampered by an over-analytical approach to her problems? Would your client be able to successfully work through her emotive issues while taking her remedies and receiving other forms of healing? Will your client be able to contact her psychological world via your therapeutic intervention?

How will you understand your client's self-concept profile?

Your client will have an opinion of herself, as a person, that may be generally favorable or unfavorable and, in either case, her self-concept will affect her healing progress. Your client may have a positive opinion of herself, perchance, may trust her own intuition and may wholeheartedly believe in herself. This will be the ideal for your client and will set her on the right foot when it comes to dealing productively with her health issues.

More often than not, however, your client will, sadly, dislike herself, will distrust her inner voice, may lack self-confidence and could adopt a self-punishing lifestyle regime. The climb for your client, in these circumstances, may be an arduous struggle and a major part of your work will, consequently, be to help her to overcome these obstacles to her success. You may, thus, need to gently persuade your client that she does have the ingredients for success, that she can act without the consent of others and that she can strive for good health for her own sake. Moreover, your client does have the right to be well, happy and healthy, despite the fact that she could often feel totally undeserving.

If your client's self-concept appears to be so poor that she dwells in an environment that might really not be supportive of her condition, or even might hamper her progress, then, perhaps, she should give serious consideration to making a positive life-style change. A punishing daily schedule, or some difficult family circumstances, may not be contributing to your client's best interests but may have arisen because she believes herself to be a doormat for whom happiness, wellbeing and abundance were not intended.

Ask yourself . . .

Does your client have a negative opinion of her health, her body and her effect on others? Will your client be caught in her own personal trap of not having sufficient confidence in her own abilities? Could your client be hampered by any lack of belief in herself and where she might be going in life? Will your client be continually dragged down by a friend or a partner who derides all her efforts to recover? Will your client be more concerned with others than with herself? Should your client be advised to take a more self-indulgent attitude to life? Can you encourage self-belief and self-trust in your client? Can you persuade your client to go with the flow of her own intuition? Does your client firmly believe that she can become her own agent of change? Might your client believe that she does not deserve to be well, happy and contented? Does your client feel that you should be concentrating your efforts on more deserving cases? Can you capitalize on your client's inherent self-belief and her determination to succeed?

How will you understand your client's spiritual-awareness profile?

Perhaps the first question to ask yourself when you greet your client will be whether she has any degree of spiritual self-awareness or any psychic ability. If your client has been readily accustomed to tapping into her own intuitive nature, and has learned to rely on this facility implicitly, then, you can often capitalize on this talent when treating her. Your client's intuitive nature will frequently put her on the right track in terms of her healing journey and will allow her to read any danger signals when things happen to go wrong. Your client, conversely, may be completely oblivious of the fact that she might possess any self-awareness faculty, whatsoever, and this factor can, then, work industriously to her disadvantage.

Almost any therapeutic intervention or any healing facility that you can render will naturally assist your client to discover and to enhance her intuitive abilities. This valuable asset will usually emerge, as if by magic, from within your client but some subtle encouragement may need to emanate from you. If, for example, your client currently resides in a state of disharmony in terms of her life circumstances, her life purpose and her immediate environment, then, her newly-developed self-awareness may, in time, rectify these areas of dissonance within her life as a spin-off from her healing journey.

Any form of therapeutic practice could, furthermore, open up your client's psychic tendencies that may have been lying dormant but are, now, ripe for discovery. Your client's belief about and her attitude towards the metaphysical aspects of her life should be carefully noted. Your client with a steadfast belief in an evolutionary destiny, a current life purpose, in multiple lifetimes, in guardian-angels and in reincarnation will have a certain mindset. Your client might, thus, place herself in a receptive frame of mind, could be encouraged to learn from life's experiences and could work towards a satisfactory solution. Alternatively, your client may believe that her destiny must be personally managed and that she will only have one chance of getting it right. Either way, both sets of beliefs can be utilized to your advantage when helping your client to overcome her ill-health, her pain and her distress. All you may need to do will be to tune into your client's beliefs about herself and her life purpose and, then, to whole-heartedly support her values.

When interviewing and interacting with your client, much ground can usually be covered if you rely on and listen attentively to your own intuition. Even if you are not an exponent of metaphysical doctrine, you can still be open to what your mind may be telling you unconsciously at any given point in time. It may, for example, be advantageous for you to note whether you can intuitively feel any ill-ease within your client in terms of energetic feedback. As a therapeutic practitioner, your intuition may be highly attuned and, hopefully, you can learn to rely on and to perfect this useful skill. By this means, you might soon be able to see, to hear and to feel your client's distress as well as being able to realize when her pain has shifted to any significant degree. If you are not yet accomplished at honing this skill, then, be assured that, with time, patience and practice, you should soon be able to read the very air itself using your intuitive powers.

Ask yourself . . .

Have you learned to trust and to rely wholeheartedly on your own intuitive powers and a higher power operating in your life? What do you truly feel about your client's condition or her state of health? What do you see, hear and feel when you interact with your client? In what ways can you utilize your client's intuitive powers? How can you further encourage your client to develop her awareness of both herself and her healing journey? Can you appreciate the ways in which your client may be developing spiritually? Could your client find a means of contacting her higher self? Can you unconsciously observe your client and learn to read the signals? In what ways might your client be way off beam in her life? Does your client sincerely believe that she alone could be in control of her destiny and her healthcare program? Will your client be in touch with her spiritual nature or will she remain in ignorant oblivion? What does your client believe about reincarnation and about spiritual evolu-

tion? Does your client subscribe to a set of metaphysical beliefs that can provide her with great comfort in times of distress? Will it be necessary for your client to believe in any spiritual doctrine in order for your treatment to be effective? Can you acknowledge your client's belief in metaphysical philosophy with glee and capitalize on her convictions? Can you accept that your client might give no credence to spiritual philosophy and still work with her accordingly?

How will you understand your client's relationship profile?

You will, of course, need to consider any significant others in your client's life when facilitating her recovery program. Sometimes the people in your client's orbit will be an asset to her and their support can rapidly aid her healing journey. Your client, alternatively, may be surrounded by those who can only be described as a dead-weight around her neck and who would contribute little or nothing to her health restoration and/or to her maintenance of optimal health.

It may be wise for you to decipher whether your client might be a gregarious socialite who loves to be the life and soul of the party or, conversely, whether she will prefer to be a solitary recluse who studiously avoids the company of others. Perhaps your client craves the company of others in order to brighten up her dull life but really she could do with her own space. Your client, on the contrary, may be too shy to venture out and to mingle with others even though this might be what she earnestly desires most in life. The main question to ask yourself, here, will be whether your client will be happy with her lot. Your client may have preferences quite different from your own but, either way, you should respect her wishes and you should attempt to gauge whether her sociability and her people-skills are adequate for her purposes.

In essence, you may seek to enquire whether your client entertains a successful, committed and rewarding relationship with an intimate partner, any close friends and any associates. You may, also, want to know whether she has a viable support-network that can assist her on her therapeutic voyage. When your client regales you with numerous tales of woe about her unhappy relationships, her uncommitted relationships and any devastating instances of infidelity or of betrayal, this miserable state may mean that you will have your work cut out for you.

Ask yourself . . .

Does your client tend to mix freely with others and does she rejoice in the company of others? Might your client prefer to be a loner and to relish her own space? Will your client be a solitary person by choice or by accident? Will your client be taking therapy for herself or in order to please someone else? Might your client dread the company of others and have poor interpersonal skills? Will your client crave company and yet she might be too painfully shy to make any friends? Would you wish that your client could get out more but, nonetheless, she may be quite content to be on her own? Will your client be in a happy and a committed relationship with an intimate partner who can be loving and kind? Will your client have a caring intimate partner who can provide her with vital support and with encouragement and who may be fully in favor of her attending your clinic? Does your client live in a climate of disharmony in which she might feel out of step with her most intimate friends and associates? Does your client have a history of failed relationships from which she has derived very little comfort and has she been left thoroughly disillusioned? Has your client ever been involved with abusive or with violent people who have misused her criminally? Does your client have any unresolved bereavement issues that she has yet to face?

How will you understand your client's life-circumstances profile?

Your client's personal circumstances will largely affect her outlook on life and naturally her health prospects. For this reason, you may wish to discover whether your client might be happy and satisfied with her personal circumstances, her work, her close family, her friends and her prospects for the future.

If your client paints a dismal picture of her life, then, be assured that things may not be conducive to her making a speedy recovery. If your client has a gross dissatisfaction with her existence, this fact alone could impede her progress and could cause stagnation in all walks of her life. Your client, in these circumstances, may need to consider carefully why she finds herself in such an unhappy situation and what positive steps she could take in order to rectify this disharmony in the shortest possible time.

Your client may realistically need to take some pretty drastic steps in order to rearrange any adverse life circumstances and, thus, to accommodate her return to good health and happiness. If financial hardship might be a major factor that will contribute to your client's malaise, then, this may not only limit the amount of therapeutic assistance that she can afford but also may preoccupy her thoughts to such an extent that she cannot entertain the prospect of dedicating herself to her own therapeutic rescue.

Ask yourself . . .

Does your client enjoy a happy life or might she be very discontented with her fate? Does your client relish her occupation or will she be hoping to win the lottery in order to escape from the tedium? Will your client be constantly struggling to make ends meet financially? Might your client be weighed down heavily by adverse circumstances? Could your client be contracted into an unhappy working life? Will your client be glued to her home because of having to care for young children or because of a lack of transport when she earnestly desires to get out more? Might your client be locked into an unhappy intimate relationship, or an unsuccessful business partnership, from which she cannot easily extricate herself either emotionally or financially? Does your client enjoy a life of relative comfort and ease and, so, can devote herself wholeheartedly to working with you?

How will you understand your client's cultural profile?

You may need to consider what your client believes in terms of her background culture and, then, mull over its effect on her health portrait. Your client may be happy with her background and her cultural programming and this, therefore, will not appear to hamper her progress in any way. Your client, alternatively, may wish to free herself from the shackles of all that she has been taught to believe culturally. Your client may, therefore, need to unwind any negative programming from the past in order to move on. It may be that your client will be required to break away from any unhelpful teachings or from any adverse propaganda before she can actually free herself from ill-health and discontentment.

If your client has been brainwashed with notions of doggedly upholding family loyalty, of impeccable social conduct and of unnecessary formality, she may be at a great disadvantage in terms of gaining independence and becoming a free-thinker. Similarly, your client's religious persuasion, if any, should be of her own making and not that imposed upon her unquestionably from a great height. If religious persuasion or spiritual doctrine can provide your client with comfort and support, then, all will be well. If, on the other hand, your client might, in some way, not be free to make her own choices impartially, then, this may be injurious to her health prospects and could constitute an obstacle to her success. The ideal for your client will be that she makes up her own mind, totally unaided, about what she wishes to believe and the way in which she desires to conduct her life as a fully-functioning and mature individual.

Ask yourself ...

Might your client be hampered by limiting cultural mores from which she cannot seem to escape? Will your client be bogged down by outmoded beliefs about social conduct or what might be socially acceptable? Does your client adhere to an unproductive doctrine just because that will have been what she has always been taught to believe? Does your client continually worry about what others might think of her? Might your client be expected to behave in a certain way with regard to her family? Does your client wish to rebel against everything that she has been taught to believe? Does your client hold strong cultural or religious views of any description that are not particularly helpful to her? Could your client hold religious or metaphysical beliefs that are a great comfort to her in all walks of life and will positively assist her healing program? Do you believe that your client might need to extricate herself from negative programming before she can begin to forge ahead?

How would your client view her adverse health?

Will your client really hold the winning ticket when on her healing path? Your client will be a unique and a peculiar animal and her success or her failure on her therapeutic voyage will be dictated by her own particular set of circumstances and her mindset that accompanies her ill-health.

How will your client view her disorder?

Invariably your client's frame of mind and the way in which she views her disorder will dictate her response to your therapeutic methodology. If your client optimistically believes herself to be capable of recovery, then, your task may be reasonably straightforward. If, however, your client might be incessantly despondent and pessimistic about success, or skeptical of alternative practice, then, this disposition will have a significant impact on her chances of winning the race. If your client does not remain confident of a successful outcome, of course, your time may need to be devoted to altering her opinion and to boosting her morale.

If your client has frequent evidence of successful progress, this may, in itself, act as a booster for her optimism but be prepared for the fact that, at any stage, she may, also, plummet into the depths of despair. Even your most optimistic client may, of course, encounter periods of gloom when she will perceive that progress has been slow and arduous. Your client may, moreover, conclude that she will simply remain on a never-ending plateau. You may be deceived into thinking that a plateau for your client will signal stagnation but a so-called period of remission may, in fact, be the time when she might really be preparing, in earnest, for her next major healing shift. You may find, however, that the darkest hour usually occurs just before dawn and a downturn in your client's outlook and her rate of progress may, in fact, indicate that she will, now, be totally ready for a change because things cannot get any worse.

It may be beneficial for you to consider whether your client has a realistic view of her condition in terms of whether her recovery program will be short and sharp or long and protracted. If your client's condition has lingered for a long time, a short-term period of treatment may be right out of the question but she may not appreciate this salient point and will often need to be subtly reeducated. The extent of your client's disorder and the length of time that she has suffered will, furthermore, have a significant impact on her rate of recovery and the amount energy that she may need to devote to her recuperation program. As always, one of your prime considerations will be to what extent your client has indulged in allopathic medicine or engaged in surgery and how long she has continued in this vein.

Ask yourself ...

Does your client normally possess a pessimistic or an optimistic outlook on life in general? Will your client be determined to succeed or will she be merely resigned to an inevitable failure? Does your client believe that a slight twinge in the back might be a signal that she will be crippled for life? Will your client be sincerely interested in helping herself or will she be a please-just-take-my-pain-away subscriber? Would your client prefer to evade recovery because she might have a vested interest in remaining unwell? Might your client think that her symptoms that have persisted for years will magically vanish overnight? Will your client's condition be a long-term chronic one that will need some considerable time to shift? Might your client have acute and alarming symptoms that have only recently manifested? Could your client make rapid progress in therapy or will she be on a slow-recovery channel? Has your client been previously wedded to the allopathic camp or will she be a dyed-in-the-wool alternative devotee? Could you take a realist view of how long it could take your client to recover in the light of your knowledge of her case?

What would be your client's attitude to self-help?

Will your client truly understand her task in the healing equation? Probably one of the first things you will need to consider, for the sake of your own sanity, may be whether your client will be prepared to put the same amount of effort into helping herself as you will devote to facilitating her health restoration.

Will your client be attuned to self-help?

If your client remains steadfastly committed and utterly determined to improve her health position, your job will be much easier and more rewarding. The greatest joy for you may be when your client will be wholeheartedly compliant with your therapeutic methodology. By this means, your client will follow your instructions to the letter, be easily guided in the appropriate direction and eventually she will take the lead in clawing her own way back.

You will, also, need to estimate the extent to which your client will actually be helping herself or, conversely, whether she might be regularly tripping herself up. If your client, generally, leads an unhealthy life, or if she indulges in using mind-numbing drugs, her road may be long and arduous, if not impossible. If your client lives a life of hardship, of unhappiness or of general dissatisfaction, the going may, also, be harsh and hard-hitting. If your client displays a quick-fix mentality, or a let's-not-get-our-hands-dirty attitude, then, your work may be a thankless task from which you could derive very little job-satisfaction. Treating your client, in these circumstances, could feel like a tedious waste of time, at best, or, alternatively, just seem like bashing your head against a brick wall. When your client appears resistant, argumentative, defensive and doggedly remains in a world of fantasy about her healing journey, she may frequently make you feel disillusioned about your mission.

Ask yourself . . .

Has your client really decided to take total responsibility for her own healing journey? Will your client be doing all that she can to help herself or might she be on a self-sabotage mission? Does your client persist in running to see the doctor when the going gets tough? Will your client be burning the candle at both ends and eating junk-food when she should be attempting to heal a biochemical disorder and to reduce her stress levels? Does your client resort to over-indulgence in alcohol, nicotine and/or social drugs when she feels the slightest bit down at heart? Are you persistently giving your client the antidote while she continues to apply the irritant? Does your client wonder why she gets a migraine when she compulsively works too hard? Will your client realize that her life has become unsatisfactory all round and that this misfortune may be adversely affecting her health? Might your client be amazed that she has not recovered but yet she has done nothing to pull her weight in the equation?

Let's take an example – Celia's story

A prospective client rang Celia one day to enquire about her rebirthing therapy. Celia was taken aback because her potential client's first question was "How much does it cost?" and her second question was "How soon can you see me?". Moreover, Celia was addressed by her prospective client as "the rebirther" rather by her name, despite the fact that this was clearly given in her advertisement. Celia, also, noted that, generally, her client appeared to be over-desperate.

Celia's reaction to this mode of approach was to feel that her client was asking the wrong questions and that, therefore, she had not appreciated what would be involved in rebirthing therapy. Celia, consequently, decided to slow her client down somewhat by asking her about her condition. It transpired that Celia's prospective client had suffered from bulimia for some time and that she was currently taking anti-depressants.

Celia realized that her prospective client would need to understand totally what would be involved in overcoming an obsessive-compulsive disorder, such as bulimia, before any treatment could commence. Celia, thus, explained to her enquirer that she would need to address her underlying psychological issues and that she would need to attend her therapeutic sessions regularly. Celia, also, pointed out to her client that taking any anti-depressants would be like washing her feet with her socks on and that this course of action would, certainly, be pulling in the opposite direction from rebirthing practice. Celia was, furthermore, wise enough to mention that drug-taking was not the answer if her client was looking for a long-term solution. Celia, then, painstakingly explained the function of anti-depressants as a means of quashing natural human emotive reactions.

When faced with the prospect of addressing her emotive issues in the present and, more particularly, in the past, Celia's client began to back off. It was, then, obvious to Celia that her client was looking for the instant cure before even taking her gloves off. Celia, therefore, carefully described the process of healing to her client, at length, but declined to offer her an appointment. Celia merely sent her enquirer a brochure and urged her to consider whether rebirthing was, in fact, a viable option for her. By this means, if her prospective client were to approach Celia again, then, she would, no doubt, have a more realistic attitude and be in a more conducive frame of mind in order to undergo her therapy.

What would be your client's expectations of recovery?

Will your client really live on this planet in terms of recovery prospects? Your client may possess many erroneous and many preconceived notions about precisely what your therapeutic practice will have to offer her.

Will your client have been fed the wrong information?

Your client may have watched the television, or read the popular press, and may have gained a completely erroneous idea of what alternative therapy will entail, generally, and what your methodology, in particularly, could do for her. Your job initially, in many cases, may be to eradicate any of your client's false notions and to provide her with a clear picture of precisely what she can and she cannot expect from you and your practice. Often your well-intentioned client will willingly grasp your point and her initial misconceptions will instantly fade.

Your client, occasionally, may not be well equipped even to understand the words that you are clearly saying to her about your work. Sometimes you may tell your client until you are blue in the face but the information will just not seep through. It will not, of course, be your fault if your client does prove to be utterly incapable of understanding the essential facts about what you have to offer her, especially when she might not be prepared to play the game. Your responsibility will be solely to impart the facts clearly to your client. Your client's responsibility will be to grasp the essence of what you are spelling out and that will be the end of the story. If your client cannot comprehend what might be expected of her, then, this will not be your cue to get out the broomstick in order to beat yourself up.

Ask yourself . . .

Will your client, in reality, be capable of understanding the essence of alternative therapy? Does your client have a misguided notion about what your therapy is all about? Is your client window-shopping rather than intending to buy? Has your client merely dropped into your consulting room out of curiosity in order to see whether this option would work for her without any real commitment to the process? Does your client believe what she might have seen on the television or have read in the popular press about your work? Does your client know only about one facet of your therapeutic discipline when, in reality, this is a very blinkered view of the subject? Might your client go about life with an unquestioning attitude? Will your client be capable of altering her off-beat opinion of your function once she has experienced a few therapeutic sessions with you? Does your client fervently expect you to perform all the miracles? Can you capitalize on your client's healthy expectation of a successful outcome?

Let's look at it another way – Going on a summer holiday

If you decide that, this year, you would like to treat yourself to a special vacation in one of the sunnier parts of the world, you might elect to book a package holiday for the summer months. With your outline holiday plans in mind, you, then, trot down to the nearest travel agent on a cold winter's day. Here you can leisurely peruse many enticing brochures, dreaming of warm nights and cool music. You imagine many exotic places in which you can bask in the glory of the sun and can laze idly on the beach, taking the occasional dip in the sea whenever the fancy takes you. The glossy brochure depicts sumptuous accommodation, resplendent scenery, glorious food and a hectic night-life. Your dreams could all come true you are told by the enthusiastic travel agent. You finally select a destination at a price that you can just about afford and, hence, you purchase your plane-ticket for paradise scheduled for midsummer.

Once you return home with your flight details and your airline-ticket, however, reality hits you. It may be cold and miserable weather, at the moment, and, so, why not bring your dream holiday forward? Down to the airport you go and demand to be put on the next plane immediately. The airport official gently points out that your flight will not be due until the summer. You protest that you have paid your money, that you have your ticket, your passport and your luggage. You say that you would like to travel, now, in order to avoid the cold and to bring your dreams to fruition instantly. Regrettably, you can only travel on the date specified on your ticket and not a moment sooner. Moreover, the weather at your chosen destination is not too hot there either right now. Would you know someone who might be attempting to travel before the scheduled flight in order to avoid the cold?

How would you detect your client's recovery pattern?

Will you be able to detect even a slight change in your client? Even when you might feel at your most despondent in terms of helping your client, be assured that something will have happened even though you may not be able to identify it clearly.

Will you ever know whether your client has undergone a healing shift?

When life with your client seems like hard work and there has been no observable desire on her part to change, do not assume that a shift has not, in fact, taken place. You may often firmly believe that you have not made any difference with your client because you will be so hell-bent on trying to spot your own failures. Appreciate, too, that you will not be able to predict, to track or to really understand your client's healing process and, therefore, it would be folly even to try. A common mistake may be for you to believe that you could ever, possibly, comprehend what might be happening to your client and, therefore, do not be tempted to tie yourself up in knots in order to stab blindly at the impossible.

When your client appears to be resisting forcibly, for example, during a session with you, maybe, you could reframe this observation by telling yourself that she could merely be acting rebelliously as she might with a parental figure. This stance on your client's part may, in fact, be reactivating an important aspect of her past experience that is, now, ripe for resolution. Your client's revisitation of her past may, in essence, therefore, become the actual key to her turn-around in therapy without your having the slightest notion of its existence.

Your client may, of course, be the epitome of skepticism, of resistance to change and of non-compliance with you and your therapeutic treatment. Your client may not report any progress and simply will cancel after the first session. This situation, however, does not spell failure either for you or for your client. The fact that your client has visited you, even if only once, will mean that something within her has stirred, although it may be hard to see this shift even under a microscope. Your client has actually made an appointment with you, has attended your clinic and, maybe, then, has decided that alternative therapy will definitely not be for her. Your client may, thus, leave in a flurry of determination never to return to cranky medicine ever again but that may not be the end of her story. If you were a fly on the wall, you might discover that your client will pick up the pieces at another time, in another place and with someone else. When this occurs, you can simply pat yourself on the back because you gave your client her first introduction to alternative practice and you allowed her to make her decision to jump only when the terrain was entirely favorable for her. Very often when your client does take flight, it will, paradoxically, mean that she has touched her soul deeply but that she may not really want to go there right away and, so, you have, in fact, done your job very thoroughly.

Do not, furthermore, be fooled into believing that your client will only make progress when you are actively working with her. After all, your client may well have made significant progress between sessions when you were nowhere to be seen. This, too, may be more evidence to support the theory that it will be your client who does the work and not you. Often your work with your client during a session will be highly telescoped and the result will be the bird falling out of the cage long after you have given it a good shake.

In all cases, your client's healing journey will show both peaks and troughs. During her so-called troughs, your client will be gearing up for her next healing crisis. Once her healing crisis has abated, your client may, subsequently, enter a period of lull when she could be making ready for the next curative wave. A seeming plateau or, perhaps, a dip in the rate of your client's progress, therefore, should merely be regarded as a time for her to prepare for the next beneficial healing phase. This situation may arise because your client will be engaging in a never-ending process of recovery, of improvement and of progression. The lull after the storm does not mean that the storm did not occur and a period of calm does not mean that there will not be another storm brewing.

Ask yourself . . .

Do you truly feel that your work with your client has not been worthwhile? Will your client be in the lull-before-the-storm phase of her healing pattern? Does your client appear to be any different, now, from the way that she was when you first met her? Does your client despair that life can never return to normality? Will your client be showing any signs of moving forward? Do you think that your client might be slipping backward down the slippery slope? Has your client's attitude to her healing journey changed at all? Can you ever be certain that your client has not made any significant change? Do you regard your client as being at a standstill and yet she believes that she has made considerable progress? Do you believe that your client has made tremendous progress, although she feels that nothing much has shifted at all? Can you detach yourself from worrying about your client's perceived lack of progress?

Will you notice your client's healing shift?

The healing shift that will follow your client's cathartic crisis can be analogous to an orgasmic experience – intensity, struggle and uncertainty before climax and pleasure. Your client's healing shift may, on many occasions, be characterized by a period of calm and stillness, followed by some turbulence that will culminate in her fight for survival. Once her crisis has abated, your client may, then, breathe a sigh of relief and, once again, her homeostatic state will return minus some of her unwanted baggage.

You may be able to perfect the art of spotting the specific healing pattern that your client will adopt. Acquiring this talent will often stop you from panicking with regard to your client's recovery rate. Sometimes your client will display an obvious pattern of movement and sometimes not. Your client may, for example, navigate a cycle of emotional crisis, followed by some physical pain, culminating in a release and a successful conclusion. Your client may, for instance, experience physical discomfort, a return of an old condition and finally some tears and shuddering before the resolution occurs. Perhaps your client will adhere to the pattern of an aggressive fight, followed by an inclination to flee and, lastly, an immobile state from which she can magically arise like Phoenix from the flames. To make matters even more complex, your client may exhibit a variety of patterns all of which will be indicative of her cycle of change over a long period. Sometimes you will be patently aware of your client's patterns but often you will not (see Figure 5.3 – *How might your client's healing shift arise?*).

Usually your client's healing pattern will occur over a number of days, weeks or months but you may be too involved in searching for the wood to see the trees. Your client may, also, have a major shift that may greatly gratify you. After this major breakthrough, however, when comparatively little or no observable activity has occurred, you may become despondent because you are, erroneously, comparing your client's past with her present. Your client, for example, may appear to freewheel for several sessions and may seem to be going nowhere. What you will need to bear in mind, in this situation, will be that your client may be riding uphill on a wave that may last some time before the downhill descent. In these circumstances, neither you nor your client could be at all aware that any change has, in fact, taken place. Remember that when your client appears to be in the throes of traveling uphill on the crest of the wave, you will not be able to see her from the shore.

Ask yourself . . .

Can you detect any abreactive and/or cathartic response in your client? Do you really believe that your client will be incapable of change for the better? When your client appears to resist change, could she, in fact, be revisiting and recreating her stagnant past? Could your client be going through hell so that she can emerge triumphant out the other side? Might your client be calmly preparing herself for a significant healing breakthrough? When your client experiences an emotional discharge, can you detect a shift thereafter? Does your client walk into your consulting room as a new person after a major healing shift? Are you looking at your client as the same person today as the one whom you once saw or whom you first met? Have you managed to detect any of your client's recovery patterns yet? Could you ever conceivably understand the way in which your client will change?

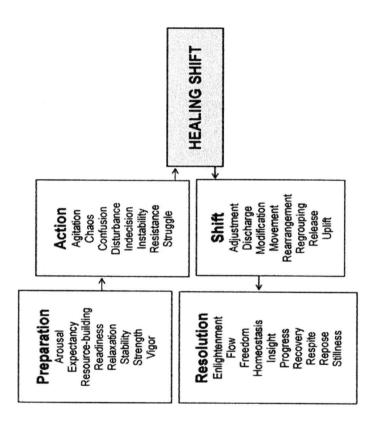

Figure 5.3 – *How might your client's healing shift arise?*

Let's take an example – Hero's story

When Hero set up in practice as a hypnotherapist, she was most concerned about the prospect of her ability to handle any abreactions that her client might experience during a therapeutic session. Throughout Hero's own training and personal therapy, she had to undergo a great deal of soul-searching in order to excise her own psychic trauma during which process she cried frequently. Hero, however, still believed deep down that shedding tears was a weakness in view of her own negative programming about emotive expression.

Hero, subsequently, saw several clients who wrestled with the inclination to show emotion and to shed tears in therapy. Hero, therefore, began to worry that she did not possess the ability to permit her client to abreact fully and that she lacked the incentive to provoke any such healing reaction. It seemed that Hero's client would arrive at a critical point but yet not have the internal impetus in order to release the pent-up emotion that would have, consequently, been cathartic. Hero believed that no real benefit could, therefore, result for her client as a result of this perceived holding back.

Hero discussed her dilemma with her supervisor because a number of her clients, who had been in this no-go situation, had failed to rebook and, so, her practice and her enthusiasm were beginning to dwindle. Hero came to realize, however, that she was making a judgment about whether her client needed to abreact in any specific way at all and whether, as a result, any cathartic change could, in fact, occur. Hero, moreover, had neglected to acknowledge that it was her client's responsibility to take advantage of the therapy on offer and, perhaps, that some delayed abreaction between sessions may well have occurred without her knowledge. Finally, Hero accepted that, in essence, the expression of tears was indicative of her client's strength of character rather than any admission of her inherent weakness. This enlightenment, thereby, released Hero from the anguish that she had experienced with regard to whether or not her client had shed tears.

6 HOW WOULD YOU CLOSELY MONITOR YOUR CLIENT?

How would you read your client accurately?

Will you be able to study your client from all angles? You should consider your client holistically as a multi-faceted physical, emotional and spiritual entity. As a practitioner, you may need to identify the links between your client's various non-disparate parts by carefully observing her from a neutral distance in order to uncover her hidden self. The secret for you will be to learn how to observe your client closely and yet from afar.

Will you see your client as others see her?

A number of therapeutic disciplines often endeavor to place your client in a given category in order to give an indication of who she has become and what her health issues might be. Because much value can be gleaned from such information, perhaps, you could investigate other practice methodology so that you can borrow philosophies from elsewhere in order to expand your own horizons.

Some basic knowledge of different holistic principles will give you an introductory guide to a number of varying therapeutic philosophies. The idea will not be for you to set yourself up in another therapeutic field entirely, or to radically change your belief-system, but merely to appreciate that a different point of view can reveal much about your client. Learning about some of the ideologies of other disciplines can often help you to see your own thinking in a clearer light. Here you can extend your own skill and, maybe, view your client from a different perspective albeit from a more secure foundation. If this preview serves to whet your appetite, then, you can, of course, stimulate it further by additional reading and further study.

Remember that all therapeutic practice will be pulling in roughly the same direction and, therefore, a peek into someone else's world could enhance your own thinking and methodology. You may notice the commonality when comparing a range of philosophies as evidence of this phenomenon. Your packaging, for instance, may be similar, or even identical, to that of your colleagues and so, perhaps, you can be invited to observe others in action.

Retain an open mind about the philosophy of other methods of practice while exploring what each might have to offer you personally and, of course, reject anything that really does not resonate with your belief-system. Despite the fact that some concepts will lean more in an entirely different direction from your particular field of work, this excursion may still be worthwhile for you in order to consider how the other half lives. By this means, you will find a way of looking at your client under a microscope without actually getting your feet wet. When it comes to reviewing your own field of knowledge, then, give yourself permission briefly to yawn and to pass on to the next section. You may, of course, entirely disagree with the facts presented here in which case remember to put your own interpretation on the data accordingly. The purpose of this section of the book will be to stimulate your own ideas and to encourage your lateral thinking. All you may need to do here will be merely to sit back and be entertained within a broad-brush approach. You may, also, find that your unconscious mind can be liberated to read your client without any conscious intervention on your part by simply absorbing the concepts highlighted below.

What would the yin-and-yang concept offer you?

Will your client achieve balance and continual change in her life? The eastern philosophy that highlights the extremes of the cosmic forces of the yin and the yang dichotomy has threads running through virtually every therapeutic discipline. Because of this familiarity with an ancient teaching, these terms of polarity have become a universal expression that can be understood even by the man in the street (see Figure 6.1 – *What might be the yin-and-yang concept?*).

Yin	Synthesis	Yang
Black	Color, grey	White
Cold, cool		Hot, warm
Chronic		Acute
Downward		Upward
Female, mother	Conception, fusion,	Male, father
Gas	Liquid	Solid
Heaven		Earth
Introvert		Extrovert
Maturity, death	Adulthood	Youth, birth
Mind, cognition	Emotions, spirit, soul	Body, physicality
Moon		Sun
Negative	Neutral	Positive
Night, darkness	Dawn, dusk, twilight	Day, daylight
Passive, receiving		Active, giving
Soft, flexible		Hard, rigid
Underactive		Overactive
Wet		Dry

Figure 6.1 – *What might be the yin-and-yang concept?*

Will your client understand black and white?

An appreciation of the symbolic value of the notion of the soft, incoming yin, at one extreme, and the hard, outgoing yang, at the other, will be a simile that rarely escapes the intelligent mind. A glance at the dichotomy principles of yin and yang will enable you to view the extremes of your client's tendencies in order, maybe, to steer her towards a synthesis in the center-ground.

As a practitioner, you will, undoubtedly, have already firmly grasped the concepts of the yin and yang within your client but take time out, now, to review these ideas with her healing picture firmly in your mind.

Ask yourself . . .

Does your client display a default tendency towards openness or towards shutdown? Will your client be focused on the emotional angle, the spiritual view or the concrete outlook? Does your client believe that her body might be separate from her mind? Might your client focus purely on her symptoms and have no notion of the fact that these may be inextricably linked to an originating cause? Does your client count her success or her progress in life from a materialistic perspective? Will your client rely on left-brain logic or on right-brain intuition in order to serve her needs? Does your client tackle life with a mature approach or might she be impulsive in her actions? Will your client be feverishly active either at dawn or at dusk? Will your client be highly stimulated and will she, in consequence, be deprived of rest? Might your client react to the softly-softly touch or will she require a more forceful and direct approach? Can your client learn to merge groundedness and practicality with creativity and spirituality? Can you perceive the yin and the yang polarities within your client?

What would the color concept offer you?

Could your client ever behold a world without color in it? The color concept arises within several therapeutic disciplines either as a tangible substance with which to work directly or merely as a symbolic instrument (see Figure 6.2 – *What might be the color concept?*).

White
Imagery Birth, clarity, coldness, naïvety, precision, purity, truth, virginity
Time/season Day, noon
Element/planet Ether, moon, space
Mineral Crystal, diamond, opal, pearl, platinum
Related colors Grey

Black
Imagery Death, elegance, formality, mourning, satanism, solitude, sorrow, underworld
Time/season Midnight, night
Mineral Jet, onyx
Related colors Ebony, grey

Grey
Imagery Calmness, coldness, neutrality, uncertainty
Time/season Dusk
Mineral Silver
Related colors Black, charcoal, silver, slate, white

Brown
Imagery Conscientiousness, endurance, fruitfulness, groundedness, practicality, rebirth, reliability, stability
Time/season Autumn, dawn
Element/planet Earth
Mineral Gold, topaz
Related colors Auburn, bronze, sepia, tan

Red
Imagery Courage, excitement, leadership, optimism, passion, power, rebellion, vibrancy
Time/season Midday, summer
Element/planet Fire
Mineral Coral, garnet, ruby
Related colors Burgundy, magenta, maroon, orange, pink, scarlet

Orange
Imagery Ambition, ardor, bravery, comfort, constructiveness, frivolity, stimulation, youth
Time/season Autumn, sunrise, sunset
Mineral Gold, topaz
Related colors Apricot, bronze, copper, gold, red, yellow

Yellow
Imagery Broad-mindedness, communication, friendliness, fun, gaiety, happiness, intellect, sunshine

Time/season Noon
Element/planet Sun
Mineral Amber, citrine, topaz
Related colors Cream, gold, orange

Green
Imagery Abundance, envy, freshness, growth, health, nature, nourishment, sympathy
Time/season Spring
Element/planet Earth
Mineral Emerald, jade
Related colors Mint, olive

Blue
Imagery Dreams, fantasy, fidelity, freedom, peace, relaxation, sea, sky
Element/planet Water
Mineral Aquamarine, sapphire, turquoise
Related colors Cyan, indigo, navy, violet

Violet
Imagery Contentment, grandeur, idealism, insight, optimism, self-respect, sensitivity, spirituality
Element/planet Ether
Mineral Amethyst
Related colors Blue, cerise, indigo, magenta, plum

Figure 6.2 – *What might be the color concept?*

Will your client paint a colored picture?

The colors of the spectrum and the colors of the rainbow are a factor of human existence and a product of the natural world that cannot be ignored by your client. Color nuances, from the vibrant and dense to the pale and virtually imperceptible, can have a profound effect on your client either overtly or subliminally.

Color can influence your client physically, mentally, emotionally and spiritually. There may frequently be hidden meanings attributed to the various colors of the spectrum and, perhaps, you can read and receive these messages that your client may be, unsuspectingly, conveying to the world. In general, the brighter colors of red, orange and yellow are believed to depict excitement and vitality, while the paler hues of green, blue and violet are usually more restful and tranquil. You may wish to experiment in order to attribute your own meanings to the various colors of the spectrum and this can be a good exercise for you in creative thinking with your client.

Ask yourself . . .

Can you interpret the symbolic meaning of the way in which your client colors her life? Might your client reflect her mood by her choice of colors in clothing or accessories? Does your client pepper her vocabulary with colorful words? Does your client complain of a black mood when her life becomes an ordeal? Could your client be in the grey area in terms of the direction that her life should take? Will an improvement in your client's condition be reflected in a warm sunny smile? Does your client earnestly seek to make her inner truth crystal clear? Can your client ground herself in reality or does she soar towards the blue sky? Could your client be purely pale and frivolous in her approach to therapeutic advancement? Could your client be green with envy or green with innocence? Does your client see red when people do not comply with her precise wishes? Does your client delight in lavender for its peace-bringing qualities? In what ways can color assist you when observing and when monitoring your client?

What would the natural-elements concept offer you?

Will your client relate to the nature of her own universe? The influence of the elements of the natural world has long been regarded as an integral part of our existence and dates back to many ancient philosophies (see Figure 6.3 – *What might be the natural-elements concept?*).

Fire
Psychology Assertiveness, enthusiasm, optimism, spontaneity, vitality
Color Red
Time/season Noon, summer
Direction South
Imagery Heat, light, warmth
Enhanced by Air
Negated by Earth, water

Earth
Psychology Analysis, patience, practicality, precision, reliability
Color Green
Time/season Midnight, winter
Direction North
Imagery Materialism, rigidity, stability
Enhanced by Water
Negated by Air, fire

Air
Psychology Alertness, communication, impartiality, intellect, resourceful-ness
Color Yellow
Time/season Dawn, spring
Direction East
Imagery Agility, expression, thought
Enhanced by Fire
Negated by Earth, water

Water
Psychology Creativity, emotions, empathy, intuition, reflection
Color Blue
Time/season Autumn, twilight
Direction West
Imagery Fluidity, inspiration, irrigation
Enhanced by Earth
Negated by Air, fire

Ether
Psychology Evolution, inner strength, self-enlightenment, self-forgiveness, spirituality
Color White
Direction Core, infinity
Imagery Space, intangibility

Figure 6.3 – *What might be the natural-elements concept?*

Will your client be at one with the elements of nature?

The elements of the natural world are, generally, regarded as fire, earth, air, water and ether each of which has both a real meaning as well as containing a symbolic interpretation. Fire warms yet devours. Earth bears fruit yet needs to be nourished. Air provides breath yet, being invisible, can unpredictably change. Water can irrigate yet swamp. Ether combines all the elements in order to form the divine life-blood of the universe. We are all subjected, whether we like it or not, to the vagaries of the weather, the climate, the seasons and the fruits of nature. From this premise, it will follow that we can relate, at least, to the symbolic meaning of the elements present in the world around us. You could experiment with the meanings behind the actual and the symbolic nature of the elements and, maybe, come up with some fresh interpretations that will be of use both to you and your client.

Ask yourself . . .

Can you put your own interpretation on your client's representation of the elements of nature? Has your client got her fingers burnt once too often? Could your client be fired up with enthusiasm or has her passion been dampened? Will your client be warm and welcoming in her approach to others? Does your client appear to be dry and barren? Has your client adopted an ice cold attitude to her emotive reactions or to her physical sensations? Does your client walk on the firm-set earth or does she build her life on castles in the air? Could your client feel stifled by life and by those in her intimate circle? Does your client attempt to outwit others with her intellect or with her academic prowess? Will your client be wide awake mentally and intellectually most of the time? Could your client be at the mercy of her own emotive responses? Does your client run roughshod over the feelings of others? Does your client consider others long before she attends to her own needs? Might your client feel that she merits nothing in life? Will your client be a damper on the enthusiasm of others? Does your client consider that she does not deserve to undertake any therapeutic healing? Does your client believe that she should improve her life mainly for the benefit of her family or her friends? Can your client readily embrace the idea of her personal evolution? Can you watch your client growing in inner strength and in personal wisdom? In what ways could the natural world and the natural elements assist you in your work?

What would the chakra-systems concept offer you?

Will you find the subtle link between your client's mind and her body? A number of healing disciplines will embrace the concept of chakra systems that can circulate subtle energies and will, therefore, govern the whole state of your client's health (see Figure 6.4 – *What might be the chakra-systems concept?*).

Root/Muladhara
Physicality Adrenal glands, coccyx, eliminative organs, lower limbs, sacral plexus
Imagery Abundance, fear, groundedness, innocence, physical identity, security, self-preservation, trust
Sense Smell
Element/planet Earth, Mars
Color Red
Musical note C

Sacral/Svadhisthana
Physicality Lumbar plexus, reproductive organs, sacrum
Imagery Appetite, dependence, desire, gender identity, movement, pleasure, self-gratification, social connection
Sense Taste
Element/planet Water, Sun
Color Orange
Musical note D

Solar Plexus/Manipura
Physicality Digestive organs, solar plexus
Imagery Anger, autonomy, effectiveness, energy, freedom, personal power, self-definition, spontaneity
Sense Sight
Element/planet Fire, Mercury
Color Yellow
Musical note E

Heart/Anahata
Physicality Cardiac plexus, circulation, heart, thymus gland
Imagery Balance, compassion, integration, openness, self-acceptance, social identity
Sense Touch
Element/planet Air, Saturn
Color Green, pink
Musical note F

Throat/Visuddha
Physicality Cervical plexus, hypothalamus, parathyroid glands, thyroid gland, upper limbs
Imagery Communication, creativity, diplomacy, fluency, grief, self-expression
Sense Hearing, speech
Element/planet Ether, Venus
Color Blue
Musical note G

Brow/Ajna
Physicality Carotid plexus, pituitary gland
Imagery Archetypal identity, imagination, intuition, memory, psychic ability, self-knowledge, self-reflection, vision
Sense Perception
Element/planet Sound, Uranus
Color Indigo
Musical note A

Crown/Sahasrara
Physicality Brain, nervous system, pineal gland
Imagery Awareness, empathy, enlightenment, self-realization, spiritual unity, universal identify, wisdom
Sense Enlightenment
Element/planet Light, Jupiter
Color Violet
Musical note B

Figure 6.4 – *What might be the chakra-systems concept?*

Will your client see east meeting west?

Healing energy can be regarded as a subtle form of rising and pulsating kundalini energy that has been variously described as the life force or the vital force in western parlance as well as being the chi, the ki, the qi or the prana in eastern philosophies. This vital healing energy, that flows within three channels of the human system, is believed to underlie your client's physical, emotional and cognitive health. This energy flow and its combined forces, therefore, will dictate your client's health and her spirituality accordingly. A harmonious and uninterrupted flow of energy, that will be neither too weak and stagnant nor too strong and severe, will result in good all-round health for your client because the chakra system will, as a result, be satisfactorily aligned and balanced.

The word chakra is a Sanskrit word meaning wheel, disk or vortex. This meaning implies that your client's bioenergy will move in a spinning motion around her energy-centers each of which will act like a pump or a valve in order to control the reception, the assimilation and the transmission of her bioenergy. A balance within your client's chakra system will be believed to bring about her self-realization and her healing zenith.

Your client's system will consist of the chakra regions that govern the lower, the middle and the upper part of her body. Your client's lower chakra region will be associated with her heritage and her earth-bound contact. Your client's middle chakra region will be concerned with her relationship with herself and with others in the social world. Your client's upper chakra region will be related to her personal evolution and her spiritual journey. The concept of subtle energy will underpin many forms of eastern medicine that will focus on your client's chakra system of concentrated energy-centers. The chakra centers will follow your client's midline and will connect to the meridian system of energy channels through which subtle energies can flow. The chakra system will correspond to your client's endocrine system and her nervous system within orthodox western medicine. In psychological terms, the chakra system will depict the way in which your client will respond to life, will form a relationship with herself and can interact with the world about her. Energetic blockages in one or more of your client's chakra regions may, in consequence, generate her presenting symptoms.

Ask yourself . . .

Can you detect which of the chakra regions are imbalanced within your client? Does your client's condition principally affect her upper or her lower body? Which of your client's senses might be most keenly alive and which has been unconsciously suppressed or been ignored by her? Could your client have security issues or does she fear for her own survival? Does your client exhibit problems of coming to terms with her sexuality and her ability to be intimate with others? Might your client be self-indulgent or be self-obsessed? Does your client depend too much on other people? Could your client be reliant on someone who has proved untrustworthy in the past yet she has not quite realized this subtle truth? Does your client display a surfeit of anger or an excess of jealousy that tends to erupt far too often? Could your client be drained of energy and be generally unresponsive? Does your client doubt her every move and does she proceed only with extreme caution? Will your client be unable to socialize and will she prefer to confine herself to her home? Could your client be afraid to speak her own truth or be unable to appreciate that she can actually be heard? Might your client be creatively blocked or be unmotivated to live the life that she would like to lead? Could your client be working towards finding her own philosophy of life? Does your client believe in her own special brand of wisdom? Could the chakra-systems concept enlighten your thinking about your client's health picture?

What would the energetic-fields concept offer you?

Will you regard your client as an integrated biosphere of energy? The human biosphere is believed to consist of seven energetic fields that can vibrate at varying frequencies in order to form your client's auric field (see Figure 6.5 – *What might be the energetic-fields concept?*).

First field
Sphere Physicality
Imagery Sensory acuity, stamina, strength, vitality

Second field
Sphere Psychology
Imagery Emotional sensitivity, self-acceptance, self-confidence, self-image

Third field
Sphere Mentality
Imagery Intuition, learning ability, mental agility, motivation

Fourth field
Sphere Relationships
Imagery Environmental interaction, intimacy, professional conduct, social alienation, social interaction

Fifth field
Sphere Divine will
Imagery Creative expression, life purpose, personal freedom, precision, symmetry

Sixth field
Sphere Divine love
Imagery Acceptance of others, meditative states, reality experience, self-healing

Seventh field
Sphere Integration
Imagery Creativity, inspiration, psychic ability, wholeness

Figure 6.5 – *What might be the energetic-fields concept?*

Will your client be aware of her own presence?

Your client's energetic fields are believed to portray her entire health picture because her personal energy and her strength will dictate her resistance to harmful stress and to invading disease. This form of analysis will, also, consider the relationships that your client may have with herself and with others as well as looking at the way in which her healing journey could evolve.

The seven energetic layers that comprise the human auric field will, moreover, emanate from and embody your client's chakra system. Your client's energetic fields will relate to her physical being, her emotional life, her mental capacity and her social relationships. Your client's personal biosphere will, thus, govern her personal space, her life purpose, her creative talents and her spiritual unfolding. Your client's sacred space will provide her with a means of fending off any unwanted invasion from intrusive outsiders when her boundaries are intact. Moreover, your client's personal space will be that part of herself that she can elect to share with others. Your client, therefore, should permit others to enter her personal space only when she wholeheartedly agrees to and desires this union to occur. If your client complains of relationship difficulties, it may be important for you to take account of any inappropriate boundary issues that she may exhibit.

Ask yourself . . .

Does your client have a healthy relationship with herself? Might your client have serious boundary issues when it comes to social interaction? Does your client avoid social interaction at all costs? Will your client have a good self-preservation instinct or do others continually impose upon her? Does your client tend to be easily controlled or readily manipulated by others? Might your client be the over-carer or the rescuer for anyone else who might be in trouble? Might your client be a habitual control-freak both with herself and towards others? Has your client ever been brutally invaded so that she has been left a vulnerable victim at the mercy of others? Does your client unwillingly permit others to dump their emotional baggage into her sacred space? Does your client appear to be alive and to be engaged in life or has she just shut down her emotional sensitivities? Could your client have any creative blockages or any lack the motivation? Will your client be stuck in a rut of hopeless indecision? Does your client appreciate nature, beauty and art? Might your client tend to rebel against accepted norms and against social conformity? Could your client believe herself to be trapped by her own emotions or does she enjoy emotional freedom and peace of mind? Does your client give you the impression of a stagnant being? Might your client opt out of participating in life and does she evade her responsibilities in life? Could your client be beset by negative thoughts and/or opinions and does she tend to rationalize all her actions? Will your client be inclined to put herself and others down readily? Does your client suffer from emotional and physical toxicity? Could your client be over-anxious about order and method? Could your client be rational or else be illogical in her thinking capacity? Can your client identify her own true health issues? Can you utilize the ideas behind the concept of energetic fields when treating your client?

What would the Chinese five-elements concept offer you?

Will you appreciate the link between your client and her immediate external environment? The Chinese five-elements system of analysis will consider your client as she will harmonize with and move through the seasons of the year and the ages of man (see Figure 6.6 – *What might be the Chinese five-elements concept?*).

Wood
Season/time Infancy, spring
Physicality Gallbladder, liver, nerves, tendons
Psychology Anger, patience
Mentality Sensitivity
Quality Generation

Fire
Season/time Adolescence, summer
Physicality Circulation, heart, small intestine
Psychology Hatred, joy
Mentality Creativity
Quality Expansion

Earth
Season/time Adulthood, late summer
Physicality Digestion, pancreas, musculature, spleen, stomach
Psychology Anxiety, empathy
Mentality Clarity
Quality Stabilization

Metal
Season/time Autumn, maturity
Physicality Large intestine, lungs, respiration, skin
Psychology Courage, grief

Mentality Intuition
Quality Contraction

Water
Season/time Death, rebirth, winter
Physicality Bladder, bone, excretion, kidneys
Psychology Calmness, fear
Mentality Spontaneity
Quality Conservation

Figure 6.6 – *What might be the Chinese five-elements concept?*

Will your client be able to capitalize on eastern teachings?

The concept of the five elements of nature can bring your client both symbolically and, in reality, in touch with the constant changes that will occur within the human system. Such changes for your client may be influenced by the climate and the ambience of the constantly changing seasons of the year. Every human creature will be affected, in some way, by the fact that there are extremes of temperature from one season to another and these seasonal differences will, unavoidably, bring forth changes in human behavior and nutritional intake.

The five elements of Chinese philosophy will relate to your client's physical, emotional, mental and energetic qualities as seen through the elements of wood, fire, metal, earth and water. An analysis of your client using the five-elements theory may, therefore, provide you with a guide to her physical, her psychological and her spiritual wellbeing. A study of this concept may reap rewards for you in your attempt to come to grips with your client's health picture at the deepest levels.

Ask yourself . . .

In which season does your client reside in terms of her temperament? Does your client consider that springtime abundance can only be reserved for others? Might your client be in a regenerative phase or else in a closing down period in her life? Can your client stop still for a moment in order to consolidate her position? Could your client be in the first flush of youth or will she display a mature presence? Could your client be in the midst of a winter of discontent? Might your client be inclined towards losing her

151

temper easily or does she exhibit a more placid and unruffled disposition? Does your client display the trusting innocence and naïvety of youth? Will your client be consumed with hatred or does she take a simple pleasure in all things? Could your client be creative and be able to bring her ideas fully to fruition? Does your client have her feet firmly on the ground in terms of being able to see it and tell it like it is? Will your client be beset by grief and yet clearly unable to get to the root of her problems? Will your client be able to bring herself to a state in which she can expand from the nub of her inner being? Does your client fear moving forward in order to generate a new life for herself? Would your client be able to trust her gut-reactions? Does your client suffer from a skin disorder that might arise during any periods of depression? Does your client make frequent trips to the loo when dealing with an anxiety-based disorder? Can you capitalize on the ideology of Chinese medical philosophy?

What would the somato-typing concept offer you?

Will you be able to behold your client as a generic being? The idea of a body-typing system that might correspond to your client's physiological condition has been encapsulated in the somato-typing concept (see Figure 6.7 – *What might be the somato-typing concept?*).

Endomorphic
Body-type Heavy-build
Appearance Plump, stocky, stout
Element Earth, water
Physiology Nutrition, vitality
Embryology Endoderm, nervous system, viscera

Mesomorphic
Body-type Medium-build
Appearance Robust, muscular
Element Fire
Physiology Movement, structure, support
Embryology Connective tissue, mesoderm

Ectomorphic
Body-type Light-build

Appearance Frail, slim
Element Air
Physiology Communication, exchange, protection
Embryology Ectoderm, mucous membrane, skin

Figure 6.7 – *What might be the somato-typing concept?*

Will your client be aware of her own stature?

The somato-typing philosophy will consider your client in terms of body-weight and build as an indicator through which to assess her overall health position. This concept can be regarded as the basis of many lines of thinking in the alternative medical and therapeutic fields.

The somato-typing concept will view your client according to whether she has a plump and heavy-build, a robust and medium-build or a frail and light-build in terms of body stature and constitution. Your client may, thus, be classified by her physical stature and appearance and this information can, then, provide you with a valuable clue to the way in which her system was formed at the moment of her conception. Your client's genetic inheritance, therefore, can intrinsically affect her health picture and, consequently, the way in which she might run her life. You might do well to endeavor to understand your client's journey through life from that moment when her being was formed and when she was merely a ball of cellular matter. It has been said that this microscopic cellular entity will hold the complete blueprint for your client's entire life.

Ask yourself . . .

Will your client be stout, be robust or be frail in stature? Will your client's stature and constitution be reflected in her attitude to life? Does your client need three square meals a day in order to generate energy? Might your client have a finely-tuned nervous disposition that will be reflected in her bodily frame? Does your client find that she craves regular physical exercise in order to remain alert and to be spiritually uplifted? Does your client have a good supporting structure in times of trouble? Could your client be afraid of contact with others in a social setting? Will your client feel small and appear vulnerable in the company of others? Does your client feel crushed by the presence of weightier people?

What would the Ayurvedic concept offer you?

Will you be able to study your client as an integrated physical being? The Ayurvedic medical philosophy has stated that your client will fall largely into a category that can indicate where her psychological and her physical health may be impaired or be imbalanced (see Figure 6.8 – *What might be the Ayurvedic concept?*).

Pitta dosha

Physicality Absorption, assimilation, digestive system, metabolism, skin, temperature-regulation
Psychology Anger, excitement, hatred, jealousy, joy
Mentality Confidence, courage, enterprise, intelligence, organization, perception, transformation, understanding
Quality Acrid, damp, fiery, fluid, hot, penetrative, sharp

Kapha dosha

Physicality Growth, lubrication, musculoskeletal system, protection, stability, storage, wound-healing
Psychology Affection, calmness, greed, patience
Mentality Attachment, devotion, lethargy, memory, sympathy, tranquility
Quality Cold, earthy, heavy, oily, slow, smooth, soft, steady, sweet, watery, wet

Vata dosha

Physicality Communication, coordination, endocrine system, movement, nervous system, respiration, sense organs, transport
Psychology Doubt, exhilaration, fear, insecurity
Mentality Imagination, indecision, intuition, resilience, sensitivity, spontaneity
Quality Airy, cold, dry, etheric, light, rough, spacious, speedy, subtle, unstable

---

Figure 6.8 – *What might be the Ayurvedic concept?*

What will your client have inherited?

The philosophy of Ayurvedic medicine will consider your client as a dosha body-type and, from this information, you will be able to deduce the likely course of her health development and her personality structure. Ayurvedic medicine would, also,

seek to empower your client by emphasizing that natural prevention will be just as important as cure.

Your client may exhibit the traits of one of the three dosha-
types and a brief knowledge of Ayurvedic philosophy will, essentially, allow you to consider all aspects of her lifestyle, her
nutrition, her psychological influences and her behaviors as well
as examining any of her disease patterns. Your client may have
a propensity towards one body-type or you may detect an imbalance in one area. By studying the concepts that underpin the
categories of this ancient system of medical care, you could reflect on whether you might glean any vital information about
your client and her overall health picture.

Ask yourself . . .

*In what ways can you relate the philosophy of the Ayurvedic concept
to your client's physical health, her emotional disorders and her energetic capacity? What might be your client's primary driving emotion
and how can she access this tendency? When your client expresses her
primary emotions, could she be touching the root cause of her disorder
or her traumatic distress? Could your client with irritable bowel syndrome be able to intuitively view her condition? Might your client with
gallstones be prepared to undergo the long process of dissolving them
or will impatience impede her? Does your client with an uncontrollable
anxiety disorder, coincidentally, suffer from muscular aches and pains?
Does your client with circulatory problems or with clogged arteries, also,
hate herself and her body for creating her disorder? Might your client
with an asthmatic condition be vulnerable to others in the outside world?
Does your client with a fear of wild animals wish to protect them from
extinction? Does your client with late-onset diabetes or with high blood-
pressure indulge in an inappropriate lifestyle? Can you see the courage
that your client will display with regard to her bereavement issues? Will
your client be well grounded, despite her difficulties with insulin resistance? Could Ayurvedic philosophy assist you to understand your client
more comprehensively?*

What would the blood-typing concept offer you?

Will you be able to view your client's systemic history back
through the generations? The blood-group analysis philosophy

will consider your client's ABO blood-type classification as a major factor in her overall health picture. Your client's genetically-inherited blood group will dictate the way in which her immune system can handle disease and how she will respond to stress (see Figure 6.9 – *What might be the blood-typing concept?*).

Blood group O
Origin Hunter-gatherers
Stress pattern Depression, substance abuse
Stress relief Exercise
Disease pattern Heart disease, Parkinson's disease, schizophrenia
Psychology Aggressive, ambitious, extroverted, hyperactive, impulsive, pragmatic, risk-taking, self-destructive
Dietary requirements Fish, game, meat, vegetables

Blood group A
Origin Cultivators, farmers
Stress pattern Anxiety disorders, phobic disorders, sleep disturbance
Stress relief Meditation
Disease pattern Cancer, diabetes, heart disease, hypothyroidism
Psychology Adaptable, anxious, cooperative, flexible, hypersensitive, introverted, irritable, obsessive, sociable, supportive
Dietary requirements Fish, grains, legumes, vegetables

Blood group B
Origin Gypsies, nomads
Stress pattern Depression, mood disturbance
Stress relief Visualization
Disease pattern Diabetes, hypothyroidism
Psychology Fluidic, idiosyncratic, independent, malleable, moody
Dietary requirements Dairy produce, fish, game, grains, meat, vegetables

Blood group AB
Origin Mixed origins
Stress pattern Depression, social withdrawal, substance abuse
Stress relief Exercise, meditation, visualization
Disease pattern Heart disease, Parkinson's disease, schizophrenia
Psychology Charismatic, intuitive, self-effacing, spiritual, visionary

Dietary requirements Fish, game, grains, legumes, meat, vegetables

Figure 6.9 – *What might be the blood-typing concept?*

What kind of an animal will your client be?

A knowledge of your client's blood group can enable you to appreciate her dietary and her lifestyle requirements as well as understanding any disease propensity and any potential stress-related responses that she may exhibit. You may well be in a better position to understand your client, therefore, if you happen to know her blood-type category so that you can ask yourself about her personality traits and her stress-response in line with blood-group guidelines. If you do not know your client's blood type, however, you may still benefit by asking yourself a number of questions about her personality traits and her behavioral motivations.

The philosophy that underpins the blood-typing concept will regard the genetic evolution of the human blood groups as mankind's inevitable quest for survival through the centuries. This system will track the genetic history of the human species back from the ancient hunter-gatherer to the latter-day modern age of man. Each of the four ABO blood groups will exhibit its own set of survivalist characteristics and, consequently, its own in-built responses to threat, to stress and to pressure from the external environment.

Ask yourself . . .

Can you identify your client's character traits and her stress-response from her blood-group classification? Does your client react in accordance with her blood-type category? Can you identify the ways in which your client has been susceptible to disease because of her inherent immune-system weakness? Can you intuitively detect your client's blood-type from her behavior and her general reactions? Would your client be an extrovert who will react well to being given a challenge? Would your client be an introvert who will warm to reflective and philosophical debate? Could your client be a high-energy person who will need to be on the go most of the time? Does your client tend to crave the quiet and the hassle-free lifestyle? Does your client respond well to creative visualization and to imaginative techniques? Might your client suffer from uncontrollable mood swings? Can you capitalize on your client's intuitive abilities and on her spiritual beliefs? Does your client appear to be a social outcast or else the life and soul of the party? Might your client be prone to depression or to substance abuse? Does your client suffer from anxieties, from fears or from phobias? Does your client tend to solve her problems by either taking action or by running away from trouble? Can you put your client in touch with her intuitive nature? Might the blood-typing philosophy throw some light on some of your client's dilemmas for you?

What would the metabolic-typing concept offer you?

Will you appreciate your client as a human biochemical and metabolic factory? Metabolic typing will be a therapeutic means of identifying the dietary and the medicinal requirements of your client. This concept will consider the ways in which your client's biochemistry will metabolize nutrients and will operate the various homeostatic controls within her system (see Figure 6.10 – *What might be the metabolic-typing concept?*).

Fast metabolism
Acid/alkaline balance Acidic
Nervous system dominance Parasympathetic
Physiology Diarrhoea, good digestion, high energy, low blood-pressure, low body-temperature, slow respiration, strong appetite
Psychology Depressive, procrastinating, relaxed, sociable
Appearance Short, stocky
Dietary requirements Low carbohydrate, high fats/oils, high protein

Slow metabolism
Acid/alkaline balance Alkaline
Nervous system dominance Sympathetic
Physiology Constipation, fast respiration, high blood-pressure, high body-temperature, low energy, poor digestion, weak appetite
Psychology Anxious, hyperactive, motivated, unsociable
Appearance Lean, tall
Dietary requirements High carbohydrate, low fats/oils, low protein

Neutral metabolism
Acid/alkaline balance Neutral

Nervous system dominance Neutral
Physiology Variable
Psychology Variable
Appearance Variable
Dietary requirements Moderate carbohydrate, moderate fats/oils, moderate protein

Figure 6.10 – *What might be the metabolic-typing concept?*

How will your client function at a cellular level?

It may be helpful for you to consider your client in terms of the way in which her system can function as a self-sufficient organism using the philosophy of metabolic-typing. A metabolic-typing analysis will determine your client's tendencies and her imbalances with regard to the functioning of her nervous system and her endocrine system. This methodology will, also, note your client's rate of metabolic oxidation of protein, carbohydrate, fats and oils that will constitute fuel for her system. Your client may, for example, be seen to process her life and her health at a fast and feverish rate, at a slow and easy-going speed or at a pace somewhere midway between these two extremes.

A glimpse into the highly-specialized world of metabolic analysis may stimulate a number of questions for you to ponder about your client. Detailed knowledge may not be important for your practice methodology but a broad-brush peek into the concept may assist you, generally, and help you to draw analogies that might be appropriate for your client.

Ask yourself . . .

Does your client thrive on a high intake of energy-packed food? Will your client be a vegetarian by inclination rather than conviction? Does your client hunger for fats, oils and salty foods? Might your client be susceptible to every bug that will currently be going around? Will your client's health be in serious decline? Does your client appear to be in tune with her environment? Does your client tend to be at the mercy of the whims of others? Might your client be immune to criticism and to inappropriate judgment? Does your client crave sweet things but, then, feel guilty about consuming them? Does your client have boundless energy or does she tire easily? Could your client be beset with depression, with anxiety or with mood swings? Can you relate, in any way, to the thinking behind metabolic typing?

What would the Myers-Briggs psychological-typing concept offer you?

Will you be able to behold your client as a psychological entity? The popular Myers-Briggs psychological-typing indicator can be employed to assess your client's personality profile in terms of the way in which she acts, she reacts and she interacts with others (see Figure 6.11 – *What might be the Myers-Briggs psychological-typing concept?*).

Energy direction
Extrovert characteristics Expressive, impulsive, sociable
Introvert characteristics Private, quiet, reflective

Information processing
Sensing characteristics Factual, practical, realistic
Intuition characteristics Aspiring, expansive, idealistic

Decision-making
Thinking characteristics Critical, objective, observant
Feeling characteristics Appreciative, participative, subjective

Life organization
Judging characteristics Closed-minded, organizing, rigid
Perceptive characteristics Enquiring, flexible, open-minded

Figure 6.11 – *What might be the Myers-Briggs psychological-typing concept?*

How will your inner client really manifest?
The Myers-Briggs system of psychological typing will consider your client's personality preferences and her inclinations that will, in turn, highlight her behavioral tendencies and her emotional traits. This psychological-profiling device can be used, in essence, to gain a fundamental understanding of your client's nature without delving too deeply into any heavy psychological categorization.

The Myers-Briggs personality profile will assess the diametrically opposed extremes of your client's personality in terms of her behavioral traits, her information-processing faculties, her decision-making abilities and the manner in which she will run her life. From this profile you could, fundamentally, estimate whether your client might be introverted, extroverted, factual, intuitive, objective, subjective, closed-minded or open-minded.

Ask yourself . . .

Can you view your client from a number of angles by reflecting on the way in which she thinks and she acts? Can you consider your client by noting the manner in which she reacts to others as either an individual or within a group? Does your client have any rigid and fixed ideas about her health picture? Does your client have a concrete and unshakeable set of beliefs about social niceties and about acceptable conduct? Will your client be open to the idea of any form of therapeutic persuasion that she cannot readily understand? Might your client be willing to have faith in her own ability to self-heal? Might your client be willing to suspend disbelief about a continually-evolving soul progressing from this life into the next? Will your client be outspoken in social company or will she become a retiring wall-flower? Might your client be down-to-earth and be practical in her approach to matters in hand? Does your client engage in life or does she merely observe without any true participation? Does your client feel wholeheartedly involved in and responsible for her own healing program? In what ways might you benefit from studying your client's psychological profile?

7 HOW WOULD YOU BE TRUE TO YOURSELF?

Would you be doing it right with your client?

Will you constantly feel threatened by the rule-book when treating your client? It may take you some time to adjust to being a practitioner and to what this strange profession will entail. Acclimatizing to your new role in life will, of course, necessitate facing your deepest fears about getting it wrong in the world of virtual reality.

Will you be taking the safe-option?

When you emerge from your initial training course with your shiny new qualification, your task will ultimately be to put your knowledge and your skill into viable practice with your real-live client. Now will be the time in which you will ply your trade and must stand up to be counted for it.

You may, quite naturally, have many misguided notions about what might be expected of you in the workplace. You may desire to deliver the perfect session to your ideal client. You may expect your client's session to run smoothly, to render the most helpful advice to her and to make a spot-on diagnosis of her case. You may, of course, expect nothing less of yourself than to administer exemplary treatment, to prescribe the magic pill and to watch your client metamorphose into a walking advertisement for your genius. You will, most probably, judge your own achievements in terms of your client's perceived success and her satisfaction with your service. If this were your thinking, then, be prepared for constant disappointment and learn to live with it.

Initially, you may well be working by the rule-book and employing a sort of painting-by-numbers methodology as a foolproof means of getting it right in practice. In the early days, especially, you may be ever watchful for any slip-ups that you think you might have made. When you first launch your practice, you may find that you have swallowed whole every single word that you have been taught by your tutors. This situation can be useful at the survival level but any adherence to someone else's doctrine can rob you of personal choice and of vital discernment when handling your client. The supposed ideal of relying on your tutor, however, cannot be utilized in the long term because, if you are constantly spoon-fed, then, you will learn to depend on another for nourishment. In order to aim to become a fully-competent practitioner, therefore, you will need to employ lateral thinking and broad-mindedness as a means of treading the path towards ultimate success. By this route, you will be able to move from ear-bashing to eye-opening as part of your professional evolution. As time progresses, and your experience builds up, you can, then, start to push the boat out more and with a degree of aplomb.

Often your worst enemy will be indecision about what action you should take with your client. There may, for instance, be a number of ways of tackling a particular problem with your client and you may feel spoilt for choice in certain situations. The best way of approaching such a crossroads might be for you to plunge in with confidence and, then, to make any appropriate adjustments for your client along the way. Obviously, if your treatment-strategy does not precisely fit your client's agenda, then, you may need to abandon your proposed scheme in favor of following her lead. You can, of course, never be absolutely sure that you will have, in fact, made the correct move with your client but intransigence will not be helpful either to you or to her. This policy alone could be the secret of your client's success and the ultimate key to your own peace of mind. Frequently reassure yourself with the knowledge that you will, at some point in your career, make some mistakes and that every practitioner before you on the planet has made several blush-making howlers and will continue to do so. When a so-called error of judgment does occur, however, you will need to take some corrective action and your personal self-awareness should allow you to hone this skill.

Remind yourself, constantly, that you are merely accompanying your client on her healing journey of which she will be the sole author and, therefore, she will set her own agenda and her personal working pace. Your client's major healing shift, or her moment of enlightenment, will arrive only when she will be truly ready and, regretfully, you may not even be there to witness her transformation. Your client's earth-shattering breakthroughs, or her deepest insights, may occur many kilometers away from your consulting room and, possibly, several years hence. Moreover, if you are going to be privileged to witness your client's major leap forward, it may only happen several sessions further down the line when she has cleared many more leaves off the track. All you can ever claim might be that you may have helped your client somewhat with the groundwork.

Ask yourself . . .

Will you be constantly looking over your own shoulder in order to see if you are performing to an impossibly high standard? Are you trying to play it safe with your client in order to minimize your margin of error? Are you concerned that you are not treating your client according to the textbook? Do you constantly assess and reassess your performance and your methods of working? Do you continually monitor your client's reaction to you? Are things simply not turning out for your client in the way in which you have been told that they should? Might your client not be having a textbook reaction or a classic response to your treatment? Can you accept that your client's progress will be her own personal responsibility?

Let's look at it another way – Landscaping the garden

Landscape-gardening is a skilled profession that requires expertise, precision judgment and an artistic flair. The landscape-gardener needs to be a designer, a builder and a horticulturalist. When the landscape-gardener elects to ply his trade, he must survey the site and will take decisions about whether the ground should be leveled, be cleared or be drained before any construction work can begin. The designer will, also, need to take into con-sideration the preferences of his client, the vagaries of the climate and the nature of the soil. First a plan must be drawn up by the designer and, then, agreed with his client before any work can commence.

Once the long-awaited seal of approval has been given by the gardener's client, a detailed plan of action can, hence, be devised. Initial drainage or site-clearance work must first take place before building the fish pond or before planting the shrubs. It would make little sense placing a Grecian statue, or laying an Italianate patio, on uneven and/or swampy ground. The gardener must, also, consider the existence of any trees that must not be uprooted, perhaps, because of a preservation order. If a tree does need to be taken down, however, then, special arrangements must be made for this work to be carried out. A tree, of course, cannot be uprooted as if it were a weed.

Building materials should be ordered, as early as possible, after an ac-curate estimate of requirements has been made. When the ground has been cleared of weeds, the gardener will not want to wait several weeks before con-struction work can commence because he simply forgot to order the building materials. Any unnecessary delay will not only displease the gardener's valued client but also will allow some fresh weeds to grow. The gardener's professional experience and his foresight should, however, prevent this oc-currence.

Plants can be obtained only when the gardener is ready to plant them and not before. A number of plants sitting on a construction-site may get damaged or may not survive above the ground. Suitable plants will need to be purchased that will accommodate the requirements of the gardener's client, the seasonal variations, the soil conditions, the sunlight, the shade and any personal design-choice. Commonsense by the gardener will usually handle this task effectively.

Everything in planning, constructing and designing the garden will occur according to the gardener's design capability, his experience, his knowl-edge, his foresight and his commonsense all of which will culminate in the creation of a most beautiful garden. A well-planned garden will stimulate the senses, will lighten the mood and should delight the beholder. Can you appreciate that you really might be an expert landscape-gardener?

Let's take an example – Mariana's story

Mariana had been in practice for a number of years as a homeopath and, therefore, had accumulated a considerable amount of experience as a practitioner. Mariana's client suffered from a heart condition and she had high blood-pressure as well as being someone who was highly-driven and, consequently, needed to take a number of medical drugs in order to compensate for her condition. Tragedy, however, struck for Mariana when her client died relatively unexpectedly. Mariana felt, at this time, that she had failed as a practitioner because she had hoped and expected to save her client's life. Mariana was, also, haunted by her client's final words to her, at her last session, in which she had stated that she did not wish to die young.

Mariana, subsequently, saw her deceased client's son, whom she had been treating for some time, but who, now, came to her for assistance following his mother's death. During this session, however, Mariana found herself telling her client how much of a failure she had felt personally as a result of his mother's death. This situation only added to Mariana's distress because she, now, believed that she had committed a breach of professional etiquette by not remaining the impartial and empathetic observer. Her deceased client's son was, however, adamant in reassuring Mariana, in no uncertain terms, that she had made a positive contribution to his mother's last years and that she had benefited enormously from her homeopathic sessions.

Mariana took her dilemma to her personal mentor, as part of her continuing professional development program, so that she could talk through her feelings and her actions with regard to her handling of these two cases. In working through this problem, Mariana came to the understanding that she had, in fact, done all that was humanly possible on her part for her late client. Furthermore, Mariana appreciated that her feelings of failure were compounded by the fact that she had recently treated a young child, who had been born with a severe chromosomal condition, from which she had died. In these circumstances, Mariana did not feel responsible for her client's death but had, still, felt very sad and vulnerable, at this time, and, so, two client-deaths in close succession had naturally disturbed her equilibrium.

Eventually, Mariana accepted that her professional misconduct was, in fact, understandable in the circumstances but, more importantly, that *dealing with this personal issue had provided her with a valuable lesson in life and had constituted a milestone in her career. Mariana emerged from her learning experience but, in future, she became acutely aware of the ever-present risk of joining in rather than remaining the unbiased observer with her client. Mariana, incidentally, continued to treat her deceased client's son successfully for several years after this episode.*

Let's take an example – Bassanio's story

Bassanio qualified as a psychotherapist who deals specifically with trauma cases for which he had received an extensive amount of training. Bassanio's initial fear, when establishing his practice, was that his client might not be seeing the best therapist and, hence, not getting the right treatment. Bassanio, also, worried that he would make a mistake with his client who might be in dire need of expert handling. Many such worries, thus, beset Bassanio because of his lack of experience in practice.

In order to overcome his fears, Bassanio decided to add to his qualifications and to continue to question others who might hold the key to his dilemma. Bassanio finally questioned an experienced colleague about how he could avoid getting it wrong with his client. Bassanio's colleague was of the opinion that many practitioners make mistakes but that his client will always get it right. This experienced practitioner, then, cited a number of occasions when she herself had made some perceived errors of judgment but still found that her client was able to make the necessary adjustments in order to pull herself through.

Bassanio took these pearls of wisdom away with him for reflection as the magic formula for his future career success. Bassanio, now, began to practice with greater confidence in his own abilities and to allow himself the luxury of making the odd so-called mistake. Furthermore, Bassanio could not always tell when mistakes were actually made and, occasionally, felt that his so-called blunders were probably not viewed as such in the eyes of his client. Henceforth, Bassanio began to gain more confidence and greater peace of mind as his experience developed and an upward success-spiral started to manifest.

Would you be doing it your way?

When will you become a trail-blazer in your practice with your client? Remember that an initial training course will merely provide a safe framework within which to work but it might not always be the unshakeable doctrine to which you should remain utterly faithful for evermore. Once you have qualified, this will be your passport to doing it in your own way in the future. Bear in mind that, as an adult, you are allowed to live by your own set of rules and not be hamstrung by the wisdom of your supposed elders and betters.

Will you become a trendsetter?

Perhaps you could consider being adventurous in terms of the way in which you might work in the future and your daring should be an integral part of your self-growth pattern as a practitioner. Permit yourself to make a few mistakes with your client, to learn from them and, hence, to move on with better insight. Convince yourself to believe that you are actually the wise one in your consulting room. Provided that you are working within the law of the land, and in accordance with professional ethics, give yourself licence to make decisions on what questions to ask your client, the number of sessions that she may require, your professional conduct, any methods of practice and any restrictions to working in a given manner. Be aware, also, that if you do not do it your way with your client, it may not work for you, at all, because your heart will not be there.

If you feel confident about working in a certain way with your client, then, be certain that this approach will be right both for you and for her. Whatever choices you make when working with your client must, logically, be right because you have elected to make those decisions with her at that time and in those circumstances. Unless you are completely insane, your judgment and your intuition will have had a reliable foundation, based on your own accumulated wisdom and on your ability to work with your client. Do not restrict yourself, therefore, by attempting to squeeze yourself into a mould created for the purposes of generalization. Being a trendsetter will mean having confidence in your decision-making abilities and accepting that some trepidation, and several understandable blunders, will all be an evitable part of the joy of evolving as a practitioner. Furthermore, if you have trained in a certain methodology and, consequently, decide that this specialty would not be for you, then, quite simply, do not bother to set up in practice in this particular field but focus, instead, on the work that you do enjoy and can excel at with ease. Consider these points about your working practices and, then, move forward without giving the matter a second thought.

Ask yourself . . .

Do you find yourself, quite naturally, straying from the accepted way of doing things with your client? Are you finding your own feet in working intuitively and working creatively with your client? Can you happily break a few rules and still act in the interests of your client? Are you forging ahead by creating your own methods and your own working practices with your client? Does your client respond to you in a unique way that suits her, despite the fact that your approach may be a bit unorthodox? Are you getting better results with your client when you let go of worrying about getting it right? Can you mould your learning or guild the lily in order to achieve the best results for your client and, then, feel happy in your work? Can you rely on the fact that your own judgment will be your best advisor? When you make a so-called error of judgment, could you ever prove that it was actually a crass mistake?

Let's look at it another way – Passing your driving test

When someone learns to drive a car, it will be important for the learner to be able to co-ordinate both physical skill and mental knowledge in line with the law of the land. Driving a car is a highly-complex skill and cannot, therefore, be acquired in one lesson. The learner must discover how to drive the car forward, in reverse, in a circle, around corners, to the right, to the left, over hills and down dales. The novice must learn to perform such feats while still keeping one hand on the steering wheel and the other on the gear-stick. The learner, too, must negotiate traffic, must stop and go at traffic lights, must drive on the correct side of the road and should avoid lamp-posts. The beginner must be able to co-ordinate directional signals and, occasionally, to glance in the rear mirror while driving along. All this complexity of activity will need to be undertaken while breathing, while listening to the radio or when carrying on a conversation with another person. The learner, moreover, must swallow the Highway Code in one gulp and be virtually able to recite it off pat in time for the dreaded theory test.

Passing the driving test will be yet another nightmarish hurdle to be overcome by the learner. The would-be driver must put both mind and body in gear in order to scrape through this ordeal and, perhaps, will need to have a couple of shots at the game. Once the much-longed-for-and-agonized-over test has eventually been passed, and the coveted full licence has been purchased, life can instantly begin anew for the driver. The newly-qualified driver must, now, learn how to drive well and truly. The fledging must flee the nest and learn how to manage without instruction or without supportive assistance. It no longer matters about crunching gears or about kangaroos hill-starts but what may, subsequently, be important will be how to survive in the everyday world of traffic negotiation and motorway madness.

The new driver will discover, at this turning point, how to please himself, how to drive in his own way and will, hence, learn by experience what may be required of being a fully-fledged driver. The new driver can break all the rules as long as he does not break the law. The new licence-holder, however, may well not drive in the way in which he has been taught at the driving-school but may, in truth, be a better driver as a result. Driving with a full licence will, of course, be utterly different from being a learner but, in future, the driver can go where he pleases. Have you passed your driving test yet and learned how to drive?

Let's take an example – Oswald's story

Oswald is a spiritual healer who decided to gain an additional qualification in craniosacral therapy following some positive experiences on the receiving end of this powerful form of treatment. On Oswald's initial training course as a craniosacral practitioner, however, he was dismayed to notice that very little reference was made to metaphysical law and almost no credence was given to the concept of spiritual evolvement. When Oswald raised these issues with his tutors, however, his ideas were not particularly well received. Oswald, then, became highly concerned that his personal beliefs and, indeed, his whole therapeutic philosophy were being disregarded and undermined.

Oswald, subsequently, consulted his own practitioner on the question of metaphysical law and its connection with craniosacral therapy. Oswald's practitioner was herself a firm believer in metaphysical law and she reassured Oswald that, once qualified, he could naturally dovetail his own philosophies into his practice with ease and by choice. Oswald was much relieved by this reassurance from his own therapist. On qualifying, therefore, Oswald set up in practice as a craniosacral practitioner with a significant metaphysical slant. Because Oswald was being true to himself and was conducting his practice in his own way, he turned out to be a very-much-in-demand practitioner who gained endless pleasure from his work.

Would your expectations be letting you down?

Will all your well-laid plans for your client start to forsake you in practice? The biggest crisis you will, probably, ever encounter, during your working life, will occur when you hit uncertainty with your client. Often what you might confidently expect just does not happen with your client. At this juncture, you may not know what to do with your client or how to cope with a situation that might have, seemingly, spiraled out of control.

Will things go according to your plan?

You may plan a session in intricate detail only to be disappointed when your client might decide that she does not wish to comply with your strategy and, so, she will take a high dive out of the window. Your perfect session with a beginning, a middle and a satisfactory conclusion has just not materialized with your client. You may, then, feel that you have seriously let your client down because your precious plan has been lost en route. This scenario may not have been what you were told about professional life while at your training school. Your panic mode may set in about the way in which you have been working with your client. Now will be the time for you to stand back, however, and to gaze at the big picture with regard to your practice methodology and your handling of your client.

When your client comes to visit you, remember that you will be working in a live situation. The session with your client will be the real thing and not the dress rehearsal and, so, anything could happen during her session. You could be at a loss for words with your client. You could discover that you do not know the answer to any of your client's questions. You might feel yourself to be out of your depth in handling your client's case. You could be mystified about how to proceed wisely, intelligently and cautiously with your client. You might find yourself showered with embarrassment or beset by frustration in front of your client. You could be so touched by your client's distress, because it resonates quite loudly with your own personal experience, that this situation will put you on the edge of tears or will consume you with anxiety. You may feel indignant about the way in which your client has been ill-treated by another or has been ravished by disease. You could be taken aback by your client's inappropriate attitude or her unfortunate manner towards you. After any catastrophic encounter with your client, you could believe that you might never want to see another customer again.

When disaster does strike with your client, however, remember that it may merely be a learning-curve for you. Calamity will simply be a part of the inevitable journey that you must take in order to gain sound confidence, valuable experience and to unravel your purpose in treading the therapeutic practitioner's path. You should fully accept that you will not, in fact, know what to do on many occasions or that your emotional state may intervene during a session with your client. Your biggest mistake, in these circumstances, may be to attempt to cover up the situation or to conceal your true feelings from your astute-eyed client. If you endeavor to deny reality at this point, your client may detect this stance and may lose faith in you as a result. If you are true to yourself, however, your client, consequently, will acknowledge and respect you as a human being and you will, thus, be able to ride the storm and to emerge triumphant.

Ask yourself . . .

Do you feel enormously relieved when your session with your client goes according to plan but become panic-stricken when it does not? Do you fear that your client will ask you a question to which you will not know the answer? Might you have a constant feeling that your client will catch you out and will relish the experience? Could you fear that your delicate emotional state will leave you feeling vulnerable and that your client will be a witness to your distress? Might you dread that your stress will reduce you to tears in front of your client and lead you to full-scale embarrassment? Do you fear getting into panic mode with your client and, then, not being able to function? Will you consider that your client could annoy you so much that you will be in danger of losing your rag with her? Do you always want your client to accept you as the wisest sage? Are you eternally hoping that you will know what to do with your client so that things can continually run smoothly? Have you discovered your personal Achilles' heel with regard to your work yet?

What would happen when you make a mistake?

How will you react at crunch-time with your client? If you think you will never make a mistake with your client, then, think again. The secret will be for you to know how you can cope with your client and with your beating heart, simultaneously, at such times.

What will be the weakest link in your chain?

You would be advised to think positively about any perceived mistakes that you might make in the course of your work with your client. When handling your real-live client, of course, life can be decidedly subjective in the alternative therapy world. In many cases, what you would consider to be a drastic error might, in reality, be interpreted by your client as a wise move. You cannot ever predict your client's reaction to you and your methodology, and you cannot ever read her mind accurately, although you could kill yourself trying.

Be comforted by the knowledge that your client's inner wisdom will always know how to put things right. Remember that it will be your client's healing journey and that she will be the only person who will actually know what will be right for her. When you do make a so-called error of judgment, then, rest assured that your client will either make any necessary adjustments or may simply not notice your blush-making gaffe.

If you practice body-oriented medicine, and fail to notice a given condition that your client might exhibit, she will soon know whether she feels relief and whether she obtains some benefit from your treatment. If you practice mind-based therapy, and make an inappropriate suggestion, then, your client will simply make the necessary adjustment in her own mind in order to accommodate her particular situation. If you prescribe alternative medicines, and you misdiagnose your client's condition, then, your remedies will not ensure her progress, or will send her in the wrong direction, and she will, as a result, be on the phone to you.

After all, the worst-case scenario could only be that your client will decide to vote with her feet. If your client does decide to reject your approach, your style, your treatment techniques, your remedies, your supplements or your advice, then, salute her for having the insight and the courage to know what might be best for her. Do not, in these circumstances, indulge in profuse groveling with your client, in sleepless nights and in self-flagellation none of which will assist either you or her. Bringing your client in touch with herself will, after all, be the name of the game and if, as a result, she might decide to quit, then, you will have succeeded in your mission and you should be proud of your achievement. There will, in any case, be no court of law that could ever prove either way whether you have, in fact, got it right or got it wrong with your client. If you maintain a proper professional conduct with your client, then, you will have nothing to fear from any litigants.

Ask yourself . . .

How will you feel when you make a so-called mistake with your client and how will you tackle the problem? How could you guard against making an error of judgment with your client? Will you ever know whether you have given your client treatment that could be ineffective? Will you know for sure when you have given your client any inappropriate advice? Can you closely monitor the effect of your prescribed supplements or your remedies for your client in order to minimize any misdiagnosis? Can you make the necessary adjustments in order to accommodate the needs and the wishes of your client without compromising your professional integrity? Can you stop beating yourself up because you think your therapy might not be effective or could be inappropriate for your client? Can you appreciate the reasons why your client chooses to consult you? How will you react when your client decides that she does not want to consult you any longer? Could you stop worrying about your treatment methodology because this could cloud your intuitive judgment? Can you ensure that you seek immediate and effective legal assistance before your client even hints at taking legal action?

Let's take an example – Ursula's story

Ursula practices a range of alternative therapies that include acupuncture and traditional Chinese medicine. Once Ursula had set up in practice, she decided to consult another more experienced practitioner in order to receive some treatment for herself. After a few sessions with her practitioner, Ursula felt rather disenchanted by the way in which her practitioner was handling her case. Ursula's practitioner used methods that were vastly different from her own working practices and, in consequence, she felt that little progress was being made.

On one occasion, Ursula turned up for her scheduled appointment, by mistake, at the wrong time. Ursula's practitioner, then, proceeded to become very visibly anxious about this error and she besought her to return at the appointed time. Ursula was, now, disconcerted by her practitioner's anxieties and she herself endeavored to render comfort to the very person who was, in fact, supposed to be assisting her. Once Ursula had recognized that she had momentarily become the guardian-angel of her own practitioner, she decided to terminate her sessions with one whom she believed to be an incompetent operator.

On reflection, however, Ursula realized that she saw her former practitioner in the role of her mother to whom she had been an unpaid counselor during her childhood. At this point, Ursula realized that she had, in fact, benefited from seeing this practitioner, with warts and all, because she had gained some very valuable insight into her own personal need to become a practitioner. In essence, therefore, one could debate whether this seasoned practitioner did, in fact, make an error, at all, just because her anxieties got the better of her when interacting with Ursula.

Will you need a crisis-point strategy?

When working as a practitioner, it may be wise for you to have a get-out-of-jail-quick strategy in order to be able to avert any impending catastrophe with your client. You should endeavor to avoid the recurrence of any previous calamity with your client by taking steps to avoid any disastrous situation the next time it could be hovering.

Develop a number of strategies for getting yourself out of any trouble with your client that will inevitably arise throughout your therapeutic career. Endeavor to expand your repertoire of escape-routes as and when you experience any difficulty with your client. You could, for example, compile a stock-list of ready-made answers to the questions that your client may pose. You could have a convenient excuse for all those occasions when your anxieties come to the fore in the presence of your client. You could find a way of telling your client that you will need to consult a reference book, or another practitioner, in order to deal with her particular case.

Always, if you can, buy yourself some thinking-time when your client poses a difficult question before you even attempt to answer it. In all sticky situations with your client, moreover, you would be advised to work through your particular dilemma with a supervisor or with a mentor, as necessary, in order to learn productively from your adverse experiences.

Ask yourself . . .

Can you happily live with uncertainty and indecision with your client? Do you have a list of stock answers to the kinds of questions that your client might pose? Can you analyze your perceived mistakes with your client and make an attempt to ensure that you can learn from your experiences? Can you predict what might go wrong when handling your client and, then, devise an effective strategy for avoiding such a disaster in the future? Could you learn to feel confident in your ability to express your views or your reactions in front of your client? Can you approach your client with confidence that will not be shaken when the wind changes direction? Could you get in touch with those anxieties that any perceived failure with your client might evoke from within you? Can you devise a reliable formula for buying yourself some thinking-time or some action-time with your client when necessary? Can you consult your supervisor or a mentor when you are in any doubt, at all, about how to proceed with your client?

Let's take an example – Olivia's story

Olivia became a spiritual healer and psychic healer and set herself up in practice successfully. Olivia's major inner fear was, however, that she was ill-equipped to do her work because she had reservations about her psychic abilities and she believed that she should be clairvoyant in order to work in a metaphysical capacity. Olivia, also, harbored a degree of skepticism about the entire philosophy of the metaphysical world, despite many occasions when her abilities were proven and her experiences demonstrated her strong psychic aptitudes.

After working for several years in the metaphysical realm, Olivia seriously considered giving up her work because of her persistent uncer-

tainty. *Crisis-point had, now, been reached by Olivia who felt that she had to make a decision about her future career because she began to regard herself as a fraud. Olivia, then, decided to confide in a colleague on this issue who was understanding and was willing to hear her confession of skepticism and serious self-doubt. By talking to her peer, Olivia was able to identify that her misgivings were, in fact, a direct manifestation of her own extreme lack of self-confidence and that this was, now, threatening to ruin her career. Olivia felt much relieved by this chance to discuss her reservations and, simultaneously, she reviewed those occasions when her psychic abilities were, in fact, patently evident. Following her discussion with her peer, Olivia felt more inclined to continue her work and to overcome her lack of self-belief. Once Olivia's personal problems had been successfully surmounted, she found that she could assist her client without judging herself too harshly. Olivia realized that she could, also, cease to worry about whether she was successful in the eyes of her client.*

As time progressed, Olivia noticed that she made fewer apologies both to her client and to the world at large about her perceived lack of ability. From this point onward, Olivia's confidence and her practice blossomed and she believed that she had overcome a major hurdle.

Would you be comparing yourself with others?

Will you be able to ditch your idyllic role-model when working with your client? A successful practitioner will be one who may simply be doing it in his own way and be utterly heedless of the way in which others might work. If you strive always to copy someone else's style, you will surely fail because you will not be remaining true to yourself.

Will you always be looking over your own shoulder?

Often looking over your own shoulder, and standing in judgment on yourself, will be your way of putting yourself down. The temptation may be great to compare yourself with another more experienced practitioner as a means of self-denigration. If you feel that you are, in any respect, an inexperienced practitioner, you may well be tempted to compare your performance with that of your former tutors or to aspire to the status of an experienced colleague who has been in practice for centuries. You may even desire to possess the competence of a well-known author in the hope that you will be successful. This ploy will mean that you are not being yourself and may be, unhelpfully, indulging in a sort of I-am-never-going-to-make-it philosophy.

Frequently, those people whom you may admire so ardently may well not be highly successful. Your hero, for instance, may be completely unknown to your potential client, who will not have heard of his street-cred or his world-fame, and, therefore, will not be seduced by it. Your mentor, for instance, may not have any success with your particular client because you alone will have gained her trust and she will, thus, have implicit confidence in your special abilities. An experienced practitioner may make it look easy because of constant practice and because of work-experience. The competent performer will appear at ease because his skill has become second nature. If you have just begun to play the fiddle, do not, now, compare yourself with a world-famous Paganini. When you have got the hang of the instrument, then, it may not matter, at all, that Paganini could be better than you.

Begin your working life by telling yourself that you have been a practitioner, and not just a humble trainee, from the very first moment when you started your preliminary training course. During your initial training course, you will have gained knowledge and acquired experience and, therefore, your paid work will merely be a continuation of that same path. If you reflect on the way you were when you first began your training program, and, then, when you first started in practice, you will, undoubtedly, see a difference. Use this form of self-reflection as your benchmark rather than tying yourself up in knots about not being a wizard. A look back into the past will, invariably, show you the way in which your methods of working, your interaction with your client, and your whole approach to your business, will have changed out of all recognition and will have naturally evolved over time.

Ask yourself . . .

Are you continually comparing your performance with that of a more seasoned practitioner? Can you find your own way of working, even though it may be quite different from the way in which your colleagues work? Are you putting yourself down by elevating someone else

179

in your estimation? Do you feel despondent because you are not getting the number of clients that your colleagues boast? Can you reflect on the way in which you felt about your first practice-client at training school? Could you compare the present with the past in order to realize how much you have evolved? Could you consider yourself as a fully-fledged practitioner from day one rather than as a mere trainee? What would need to happen for you in order to prove to yourself that you can do it well?

Let's take an example – Helena's story

Helena very much wanted to become a hypnotherapist as her chosen occupation following a successful training course. Helena, however, just did not seem to be able to get started in her work because she harbored an extremely crippling fear of failure. Helena believed, for instance, that any established or any qualified practitioner would be fully accomplished and, so, she came to the conclusion that she did not have what it takes to match up to the competition. Moreover, Helena personally consulted a practitioner, in her own field, and felt very insignificant in the presence of this revered expert.

Helena, then, began talking to other practitioners and to fellow-trainees who had taken the plunge and who had started in practice. Helena soon realized, from these discussions, that the key to her dilemma would be, firstly, to ease herself gently into working professionally and, secondly, to take a detached view of her own performance. Helena, thus, decided to see only a few clients with whom she felt extremely comfort-able and not to accept anyone who, in any way, sounded aggressive or appeared over-confident. Helena, furthermore, spent much time in telling herself that she was not personally responsible for what her client was able to achieve but was merely doing her job as a catalyst for change. The onus for her client's healing was, therefore, taken off Helena's shoulders and placed firmly and squarely where it belonged – at someone else's door. This change of emphasis, in consequence, allowed Helena to relax sufficiently and to tentatively get started in practice and not to become over-concerned with what her client was doing.

Would you truly be a catalyst for your client?

Will you have what it takes to set the world on fire when assisting your client? The very best claim that you could ever, realistically, make, within any form of healing discipline, will merely be to assist your client on her personal healing journey.

What will you realistically offer your client?

You can never truly cure, remedy, fix or heal your client, although you can lay the turf and, then, hope that it will grow, provided, of course, that she agrees to water it. This notion should never leave your thoughts when interacting with your client. Your client alone must do the work while you just purely watch, encourage, facilitate, guide and act as a vehicle through which she may take the opportunity to improve her own health. The principle that you can only ever, at best, be a catalyst for your client should keep you stone-cold sober and ensure that you can walk in a straight line.

This news may, unfortunately, be received with great disappointment by your client who may have a vested interest in regarding you as the magic curer of all ills. You will need, in these circumstances, to keep your feet firmly on the ground and your head clear in case your client should reside in cloud-cuckoo land. When you encounter the wishful-thinker, it will pay you to bring your client down to earth rapidly with a bump in order to ensure that you do not get sucked into the trap of losing sight of the purpose of your therapeutic intervention.

Do not, in any way, set yourself up as a sorcerer because you will surely regret it and obviously will not yet have discovered your true role as a practitioner. Once your client has made the decision to improve her own health condition, and has agreed to follow your guidance, then, success may be her prize in terms of health improvement, restoration and maintenance but no guarantee can ever be given by you or anyone else in the world. The reward that your client will receive for her dedication and her effort may be optimal wellbeing, longevity, heightened self-awareness and fulfillment of her potential in life. Your client's renewed vigor may affect many future generations but she will be the only person to be congratulated on these achievements because you can really take very little credit.

Ask yourself . . .

Does your client truly understand her role in the proceedings? Will your client be inclined to believe that you must be a miracle-worker? Could your client be putting herself down by hero-worshipping you? Could your client be attempting to evade her personal responsibility by promoting your role in the equation? Are you flattered when your client praises your abilities? Can you encourage your client to feel praise for her own achievements? Do you feel that all the credit must be due to you for your client's successful recovery process? Could you simply allow your client to get on with her work and just nudge her in the right direction occasionally?

Let's take an example – Graziano's story

Graziano is a practising homeopath who had built up a sturdy repu-tation and who had stacked up many years of experience. Graziano was approached one day by a homeopathic student who enquired whether he felt that it was, in fact, necessary for her to receive homeopathic treatment personally. The homeopathic student had been advised by her training organization that she should receive some personal therapy. The stu-dent, however, wondered whether this might be a waste of money and, so, asked for Graziano's opinion. Obviously, the homeopathic student understood that she would need to experience the homeopathy that she intended to practice but resisted the idea of taking a full-length course of treatment because she considered herself to be in excellent health.

Graziano explained that, in fact, he had personally learned more about treating others by undergoing homeopathic therapy himself than he had from any training course that he had undertaken. Graziano men-tioned that he had received an extensive amount of training but that he had become skilled in the job by learning about himself and the subtle way in which homeopathic remedies can assist both mind and body heal-ing.

Graziano, also, pointed out that any prospective client will usually have more confidence in someone who has personal experience of treat-ment as well as possessing a thorough training and, therefore, spending money on personal therapy should be regarded as an investment rather than as a frivolous waste of financial resources. Graziano, in addition, explained to his bemused student-client that taking personal therapy will often give a practitioner an edge over the competition because she can, then, become a fully-rounded person to whom her clients will, synchronistically, be attracted. Graziano, finally, asked the student what she would do if she had to have a tooth extracted. Would she prefer to consult a professionally-qualified dentist who might be able to provide a painless extraction? Or would she merely tie one end of a piece to string around her tooth and the other around the door handle and, then, ask a friend to close the door on the way out?

Would you be taking note of your own performance?

Will you be able to throw away the calculator when treating your client? You may be tempted to judge yourself by results and, therefore, you will count only your perceived successes or, conversely, just your obvious failures.

Will you become an impartial observer of your own actions?

The temptation to preen your feathers when your client improves her condition magnificently may be overwhelming but you might be advised to resist this dangerous attraction. When your client turns out to be a complete failure in your eyes, however, your professional self-esteem may, then, take an unpleasant nosedive once you have succumbed to the appeal of praising yourself for perceived success.

As a practitioner, remember that you cannot be either a success or a failure because only your client can attain those privileges. For your own stability of mind, your best course of action will be to steer the middle ground in terms of your opinions of your client's progress. Be neither elated when your client succeeds nor despondent if she fails. Indeed, be interested and be delighted for her when your client achieves her objectives but do not judge yourself, in any way, by her perceived success or any lack of it. Remain a detached and an impartial observer so that your emotions and your self-esteem will not take a constant roller-coaster ride at the dictates of your client's perceived health picture.

You may be unique in that your client will elect you as her sole charioteer. Your reticent client, for example, may not have had the wherewithal to achieve success with another practitioner. Despite this apparent evidence of your prowess, still remember that you are only the catalyst and not the converter with your client. The best you could ever, possibly, hope for may be simply to be a good activist but not a miracle-worker with your client. Maybe on a good day you could permit yourself a quiet pat on the back, once your client is well and truly out of sight, but always bear in mind the fact that you are a third-party facilitator and not the instigator of her success.

Ask yourself . . .

Do you truly believe yourself to be a catalyst for change with your client? Are you ever tempted to feel overly proud when your client praises your achievements? Do you dread the fact that your client will not get better because her lack of success will dent your self-image? Can you become an impartial observer of your client's progress without becoming intimately or emotionally involved? Do you truly believe that your client would not have made it without you? How would you feel if your client believed that you were the sole key to her recovery? Are you truly happy for your client when she succeeds? Do you feel despondent when your client appears to question your methodology? Do you feel dismayed when your client reports that she has made little or no progress lately? Do you expect your client to have a major healing shift every time that she sees you? Can you avoid the disaster-trap of believing that your success must be, inextricably, bound to your client's opinions of her own progress?

Let's look at it another way – The mince-pie factory

At Christmas time there will be many mince-pies in the shops. Mince-pies are traditional Christmas goodies and the food-market will encourage and pander to such a convention in the hope of selling many packets of mince-pies. In the festive period, mince-pie factories will be working overtime in order to produce crates of these seasonal delicacies. Shops will devote whole shelves to a variety of products that will tempt the hungry festive-shopper. There will be mince-pies for brandy-lovers, for those with a sweet-tooth, for weight-watchers and for vegetarians.

The mince-pie maker may have perfected his art over many years and will know expertly how to make the tastiest of Christmas fayre. The mince-pie maker will know just how many currants and how many raisins to use in the recipe, precisely how much brandy to add and whether candied peel or suet will enhance the flavor. But the mince-pie maker will not be concerned with those consumers who do not actually like mince-pies. The mince-pie maker will not be interested in those people on a strict wheat-free diet, on

184

an anti-candida regime or those who religiously abstain from alcohol. The mince-pie maker will not be catering for those people who would prefer sausage rolls or shortbread. The mince-pie maker will care not a whit whether the purchaser might have cream or brandy butter with the product.

The mince-pie maker cannot be held responsible, in any way, for the fact that mince-pies may, at a whim, go out of fashion in favor of Danish pastries or cheese straws. The only concerns for the factory-owners will be whether production will need to switch to another commodity because the fashion in mince-pies has declined or because the media have fabricated a health-scare. As long as seasonal mince-pie-eating prevails, the mince-pie factory will be concerned only with meeting the tastes and the preferences of the market.

The quality-control manager will, of course, take the stick if somehow sausage-meat creeps into the produce rather than mincemeat but this error may be the only real cause for concern. Simply predicting the market, sticking to or improving on the time-honored recipe, and getting the goods out on time, may be all that will be required in order to satisfy the demands of the seasonal market. The man on the factory-floor does not blame himself, or hold himself responsible, for the whims of the public's tastebuds. The Christmas shopper is the one responsible for making a choice about what he wishes to eat during the festive season. What will you eat at your next Christmas feast?

Let's take an example – Hermia's story

Hermia, a flower essence practitioner, worried a great deal about being too judgmental with her client because it had been a stance that had been strongly condemned on her training course. Hermia was, therefore, concerned about any opinions that she might form about her client because this could, in some way, interrupt her progress. Hermia, consequently, sought to examine her own motivations in this respect.

Hermia, of course, appreciated that she would need to make an assessment of where her client was coming from in order to be able to prescribe a specific remedy but wondered whether she had become over-enthusiastic about character-labeling. Hermia might believe, for instance, that her client was not prepared to help herself or was not going to make any real effort to improve. These conclusions would, then, inevitably influence Hermia's decision-making and her approach to her client.

When discussing this dilemma with a colleague, Hermia realized that she was putting too much of a strain on herself by judging herself and her performance too harshly. Hermia, moreover, realized that some of her clients were, in fact, not prepared to play ball and were consummate time-wasters. When Hermia examined her personal background during meditation, she realized that she had a history of feeling obliged to always get it right. Hermia was constantly compared to others in childhood and made to feel inferior by her mother. "Could do better" was invariably written on Hermia's school report and this adage had been taken to heart by her. Thus, Hermia realized that she was, in fact, judging herself too severely and that she should start to be nice to herself instead. Hermia, in addition, elected to gently disengage herself from any client who was malingering or only window-shopping so that she could focus solely on those who were prepared to run the extra mile.

8 WOULD YOU HAVE FACED YOUR INNER DEMONS YET?

When would you meet your inner demons?

Who will be your worst critic, judge, jury and hangman in the course of your healing work with your client? Often the road to becoming a therapeutic practitioner will not be exclusively smooth and blissful and coming to terms with this disheartening fact may entail some soul-searching and some heart-rending on your part.

When will you quake in your shoes?

You may be beset by many feelings of insecurity that may arise like an army of inner demons whose sole endeavor will be to haunt you perpetually while working with your client. Evolving as a practitioner will entail recognizing, living with and, hopefully, even banishing some of those menacing goblins. A thankless task, perhaps, but actually your only means of survival in your endless quest for job-satisfaction and effective self-growth.

There can be no shame in having inner demons because they simply need to be heard, acknowledged, understood and persuasively invited to leave the arena. There will, of course, be a danger to yourself and to your client in denying that your inner demons exist. Banishing your demons will be a natural, and often an inevitable, part of your self-growth program and this path will, almost certainly, be the reason why you have embarked on becoming a healing practitioner in the first place. If you are a newly-qualified practitioner, then, you may find that you will have millions of demons lurking deep inside. If you are a seasoned practitioner, however, the only difference may be that you will have become more acquainted with your special enemies. To be a successful and a dynamic practitioner who can sleep easily at nights you will, without question, need to face your personally-assigned tormentors certainly quite regularly, if not on a daily basis.

Ask yourself . . .

Are you terrified of making a serious oversight with your client and will you greet her at every session with much trepidation? Will your sleep be disturbed by your client because you, inadvertently, get drawn into your deepest fears about being an effective practitioner? Do you live in dread of the fact that your client may find your weakest spot? Do you suspect that you will fall flat on your face with your client at the slightest provocation? Are you consciously trying hard to maintain a professional persona with your client? Do you feel yourself to be desperately over-anxious to get it right or over-eager to please your client? Could you find that when your guard might be down and you feel safe, your client will, then, suddenly tie you up in knots? Would you feel that you know nothing about your profession and that you might be unable to carry out your function as a professional? Do you consider that you lack the motivation to be able to advertise your services or to book an appointment for your prospective client?

Let's take an example – Miranda's story

Miranda took a number of years to train as a rebirthing practitioner and she dragged her coat frequently when it came to completing her course work. Miranda attributed her intransigence to the fact that she really did not want to face her own childhood issues. Miranda, also, feared that her long-standing depressive disorder would affect the work that she intended to do with her client and, so, she was slow in starting up her business even when she did eventually qualify. Miranda felt that her own personal issues would be triggered by her client's problems and that she would, then, be unable to cope with her resulting psychological upheaval. Miranda, moreover, feared that her own distress would have a knock-on effect on her family and her home-life.

Miranda, generally, felt that she was not really equipped to treat any client who had suffered from a violent or an abusive upbringing, despite the fact that she herself had been obliged to suffer from a similar start in life. When treating her client with a problem similar to her own, Miranda would, consequently, become over-anxious about getting it absolutely right. Miranda, therefore, was forced to work diligently through her own issues for some time in supervision.

Finally, Miranda came to the conclusion that she should, now, focus on the success of her client rather than dwelling on her own perceived inadequacies. Miranda, thus, reflected on the number of referrals that she had received from satisfied clients whom she had, in fact, assisted successfully with some very traumatic problems. Miranda, also, decided to help herself by continuing with her personal therapy and making sure that she talked freely to her colleagues. Miranda, of course, began to realize that part of her mission in life would be to take care of herself while working in such a specialized area. Miranda resolved, therefore, to allocate herself regular relaxation periods, to exercise regularly and to plan holidays because she appreciated that she could easily get into the downward spiral of being an over-dedicated professional.

Miranda struggled with her finances in the early stages and was concerned that she could not continue in practice because she was initially not making enough money. Miranda found a means of overcoming this hurdle, however, by taking a part-time job that bridged the financial gap and allowed her to continue with the work that she, now, greatly enjoyed.

Would you enjoy working with your client?

Will you be letting yourself down by letting your client get away with murder? Whenever you feel in the least unhappy about working with your client, for any reason at all, then, you owe it to yourself not to do so. When your client has become hard to handle, taxes your stamina, or otherwise tries your patience beyond endurance, your job-satisfaction may take a plunge and this situation will disturb your equilibrium and, therefore, you may need to take some rectifying action.

Will your client be right for you?

If you find that your client has become too tiresome or too problematic to deal with, for whatever reason, then, the solution will be simple – do not treat that customer. You do not have an inescapable obligation as a practitioner to deal with any client who demands your services. You may find that you are doing yourself a great disservice if you are attempting to handle any client who may give you little or non-existent pleasure purely because you think you may have a bounden duty to do so.

Do not let the tail wag the dog just because you are in a caring profession. You are not designed to do the impossible merely because there may be many people out there who may be in need of some therapeutic assistance. An I-must-sacrifice-myself strategy will be self-defeating both for you and for your client and this eventuality should be avoided at all costs. If it will not work for you, then, be assured that it will certainly not work for your client. You may elect to refer your client to another practitioner, or else point her in the right direction, but you are allowed to say "no thank you" when it suits you for no obvious reason at all.

Ask yourself . . .

Can you assess whether you are truly willing and able to treat your prospective client? Do you believe that you do not wish to work with your prospective client but cannot particularly explain your reaction? Might you feel out of your depth with your client whose case seems beyond your competence and your experience? What might your intuition be telling you about your prospective client? Do you believe that you have a heaven-sent duty to treat any prospective client who cares to contact you? Could you harbor a strange belief that you have been assigned a special mission to heal the masses? Do you fear having to say "no" and having to be firm about it with your client? When your client becomes a strain, are you able to bring her sessions with you to an abrupt end, if necessary?

How will you gracefully decline your client?

It will not be obligatory for you to deal with your client if you feel unqualified to do so or, in any way, uncertain about treating her just because she knocks at your door. Put job-satisfaction at the top of your own agenda and protect your comfort-zone, at all times, with regard to treating your client. Be kind to yourself and, certainly, do not stack up trouble for yourself in the course of your work. If your client demands too much of you, if she appears to have little appreciation of what your methodology might entail, or if, in any way, she might indicate that she may be becoming extremely hard work, then, give yourself permission to decline to continue to treat her. Failure to decline any unwanted client, or to deflect any existing redundant client, will be making a rod for your own back. If you act against your inner wishes with your client, you will be seriously compromising yourself and you may well regret the consequences of your actions.

Listen to your intuition that will tell you whether or not you will enjoy working with any prospective client. Give yourself the benefit of the doubt and not your prospective client. If you are in any doubt whatsoever about accepting your client, then, the best course of action will be for you to refuse to see her just in case things do go awry for you. In these circumstances, you should decline to accept your client into your practice up front, although you could, if you wish, refer her to another practitioner. It will, of course, be much easier for you to decline any prospective client immediately than it would be for you to have to ask her to leave, at a later date, when matters might have got totally out of hand.

If your existing client has proved too challenging, moreover, and you have decided that you can no longer treat her, simply refer her to another practitioner by definitively telling her that you cannot assist her any further because her healing process with you has been completed. All you can ever be expected to do will be to move your client further along the road either with your assistance or with that of another practitioner. Think out your wording carefully before you address your client and do not begin or end your speech with an apology. Sometimes, it may be sufficient for you simply not to offer her any further appointments. When you get out of your depth well and truly with your client, of course, you may need to contact your supervisor or your mentor.

On those occasions when you might feel uncomfortable with your client for no discernible reason, however, you may find that this situation will be guiding you towards self-investigation. When you feel afraid to venture into a given territory, then, do yourself a favor and do not put yourself in the lion's den. Alternatively, you could bite the bullet and face your dilemma by retaining your client and, simultaneously, endeavoring earnestly to work through your personal impasse with her. At this point, of course, you would be advised to consult your supervisor for assistance. By this means, you can often work through your inhibitions by investigating the reasons why you are so reticent about dealing with a certain condition, or getting yourself into a confrontational situation, with your client. If the situation reaches a point beyond redemption, then, declining point blank to continue treating your client, and, perhaps, referring her to another practitioner, may be your only feasible option. If the situation with your client can be retrieved, however, then, you will need to tread very carefully in order to ensure that you do not suffer personally because of your dilemma.

Ask yourself . . .

Do you get that uncomfortable feeling when your client might be due to see you? Are you over-stretching yourself because you feel that your client desperately needs you or has become dependent on you? Do you feel uneasy all the while your client is in your presence and are you very much relieved after she has left? Do you dread the fact that your client might ring up between sessions and could catch you on the back foot? Does your client have a knack of putting you on the spot and making you feel out of control or feel uncomfortable? Are your inhibitions about working with your client real or imagined? Did you fail to listen to your intuition when working with your client and are you, now, beginning to regret it? Could you overcome your problems with regard to working with your client by seeking outside advice and assistance in order to get you over the next hurdle? Have you worked out, in detail, how to tell your prospective client that you cannot treat her? Can you rehearse a speech that will leave your client in no doubt at all about the fact that you cannot see her again? Can you discuss your dilemma, and your escape-route tactics, with a colleague, a mentor or a supervisor if you wish to terminate your client's sessions with you?

Let's take an example – Ophelia's story

Ophelia is a craniosacral therapist who was treating an elderly pensioner with whom she encountered a major difficulty. When administering her therapy, Ophelia was disturbed by the fact that her client began to talk openly about his amorous encounters with women. Despite the fact that Ophelia's client was not vulgar or obscene, in any way, she, still, felt uncomfortable about listening to this aspect of his life. Ophelia, moreover, felt personally compromised and uneasy about this situation and she considered that it was inappropriate for her to have to listen to her client's thoughts in this way. Ophelia believed that her client was making a pathetic effort to exploit the intimacy of the therapeutic setting for his own ends and she, therefore, felt powerless in this situation.

Ophelia was able to work through her predicament with her supervisor who highlighted the potential pitfalls of her discomfort in this situation. Ophelia, then, decided that she would discontinue her sessions with her client. At the end of the next session, therefore, Ophelia openly told her client that his next appointment would need to be with a fellow, male colleague in her clinic because she was not able to see him any longer. Ophelia felt empathetic towards her client and his distress but did not, in any way, wish to further compromise herself.

When leaving the consulting room on this last occasion, Ophelia's client asked her for a kiss that she obviously declined. When Ophelia's client began to argue his case, she felt threatened and eventually, albeit reluctantly, submitted to a peck on the cheek as a means of getting him out of her consulting room in the shortest possible time. Ophelia, now, felt enormously relieved because she would no longer need to deal with such a difficult and embarrassing customer.

Let's take an example – Hermione's story

Hermione works as a reflexologist who specializes in offering techniques that she has developed herself in order to assist women with fertility and hormonal balance. By using reflexology in this way, Hermione has successfully assisted many women to conceive naturally, to have an easy pregnancy term and to achieve a trouble-free labor.

Over the course of time, however, Hermione began to find that when treating a woman who was simultaneously undergoing any form of in vitro fertilization (IVF) treatment, her client would achieve little or no success. Hermione was, therefore, not gaining the job-satisfaction that she had come to expect with such cases. Hermione soon began to feel that IVF methodology was at such variance with a woman's innate ability to conceive that reflexology, as a natural route to fertility, in such cases, would not prove worthwhile. Hermione came to the conclusion, therefore, that medical intervention would be pulling so far in the opposite direction from her own work that she could offer no significant hope to any client who wished to take the medical route, even though a reflexology session would, still, afford her some time to talk and to relax. In contemplating this dilemma, Hermione came to the realization that any prospective client who was undergoing IVF interventionist treatment was, in fact, at the opposite end of the spectrum from that of conceiving naturally with the aid of reflexology.

Hermione, henceforth, began to provide her prospective client with the true facts about natural fertility. Hermione, also, made a positive move to decline any potential client who would not be prepared to tune into her own system and to enhance her natural sensitivities to hormonal fluctuations in order to aid her conception.

Would you be compromising yourself?

Will self-care be placed at the top of your personal agenda when treating your client? Before you even attempt to care for your client, you must remember to look after yourself. This may appear to be a contradiction in terms for someone working in the caring profession but failure to comply with this sacrosanct rule could result in catastrophe for you and for your professional life.

Will you be burning yourself out?

Working as a practitioner may be the one time in your life when you should learn to be selfish and aim to look after yourself. When you care tirelessly for others, there may be an inevitable price to pay. The well-known danger signals for the burnout-syndrome for you will be overwork, overwhelm and over-the-top devotion to duty. If you see too many clients and you work late hours, then, you will inevitably feel the pinch. If you squeeze just another client into your already-tight schedule when you are really over-stretched, she will suffer because you will not be on your top form. If you unstintingly work yourself into the ground in the name of being a virtuous healer, then, you will be heading for disillusionment. If you work when you are tired, or you should be on holiday, then, you will become over-exhausted and inefficient. If you go out of your way to be too obliging to your client, over and above the call of duty, you may feel unappreciated and/or put upon.

If you seek to prostrate yourself, in any manner, for the benefit of your client, then, you will not be doing yourself a favor and this self-imposed pressure will, undoubtedly, affect you and your entire client-base. If you run yourself into the ground as a caring professional, you will suffer from poor performance, frustration, despondency and disenchantment. Your own health may suffer as a result of your over-devotion to duty and this will not assist your client at all. If you think you are indispensable, then, revise your thinking before it could be too late. Do not be in denial about your personal needs and your wishes as, now, will be the time to practice what you preach.

One way of guarding against the danger of any burnout-syndrome will be to ensure that you have a robust support-network. For this reason, it may not be false economy to employ a supervisor on whom you can regularly unload. Moreover, if you have a network of colleagues with whom you can discuss your own personal problems, particularly when your work begins to affect your equilibrium, then, this will be a priceless and invaluable asset for you. When you help yourself, you will, by implication, be helping your entire clientele and all those in your sphere of influence.

Ask yourself . . .

Can you detect your own personal burnout-syndrome tendency and can you guard against this possible occurrence in future? Are you ever tempted to take on too many clients and to work yourself into the ground? Can your client put subtle pressure on you in order to gain an extra pound of flesh from you? Might there be one day or one evening when you feel that you are working extra long hours? How do you perform with your client when you are over-tired or when you are unwell?

Do you believe that you are on a special healing mission with your client for whom you will need to make some personal sacrifices? Do you have a self-punishing attitude towards yourself when treating your client?

Let's take an example – Cleopatra's story

Cleopatra is a practising counselor and hypnotherapist who is able to offer a wide range of therapeutic techniques to her clients. Cleopatra began working with her client who reported having fantasies of killing himself and his family members. During her initial case-study interview with her client, Cleopatra asked him if he had been taking any medication during a period when he stayed in hospital. Cleopatra's client admitted that he had taken medication for a limited period of time but was evasive when asked to name the actual drug that he had been administered. Cleopatra's client claimed that he had been disillusioned with orthodox psychiatric treatment and, now, wanted to tackle his problems in a holistic manner. Cleopatra, however, insisted that her client provide her with the name of the drug that he had taken in view of the nature of his presenting symptoms.

At his next session, Cleopatra's client revealed the name of the drug that he had been prescribed while in hospital. Cleopatra was, consequently, able to identify the fact that her client had been prescribed an anti-psychotic drug. Cleopatra, of course, now, felt uncertain about working with her client using hypnosis because of the form of medication that he had received in the past. Cleopatra believed that treating a psychotic client with hypnosis was, possibly, inappropriate and would, in any case, have contravened her professional code of ethics.

At this point, Cleopatra was able to keep calm and to draw clear boundaries for herself and her client. Cleopatra, tactfully, explained her position to her client and pointed out the fact that she did not want to put her own professional reputation on the line. Cleopatra did, however, agree to work with her client using stress management counseling techniques that would allow him to manage his lifestyle and to cope with his stresses. Cleopatra's client was, thus, given some very useful tools in order to manage his problems but he did not undertake any in-depth psychotherapeutic investigation that might have carried a built-in risk of psychological disturbance during his healing crises.

Essentially, Cleopatra had stood her ground in insisting that she be fully informed about the form of medication that her client had taken and, because she had felt uneasy about the situation, she had wisely decided not to compromise herself. Cleopatra had been able to successfully renegotiate her working basis with her client and, thus, both parties were satisfied and were accommodated without any inherent dangers either to client or to practitioner.

How would your client react to you?

What will your client discover about herself when working with you? A knowledge of the way in which relationships can work will be a vital component of your survival-kit in the therapeutic world. It may be essential for you to understand the way in which your client could respond to you, as the custodian of her wellbeing, and for you to learn how to handle her reactions appropriately. Be assured of one solid truth – your client will think irrational things about you and you will think illogical things about her.

Why will you press your client's buttons?

The key to understanding your client's relationship with you will lie within the phenomenon known as transference. Therapeutic transference will occur because your client will, quite unconsciously, project her emotional baggage, obtained from significant others in the past, on to you in the present (see Figure 8.1 – *How might transference arise with your client?*).

Therapeutic transference can occur in any form of clinical encounter with your client, whatever your practice methodology, and will not be the exclusive domain of the mind-oriented practitioner. Transference will usually arise from within your client because your close and confidential relationship with her, in the present, will remind her of her intimate relationship with one or more significant others from her past. The therapeutic atmosphere will be the ideal breeding ground, therefore, for your client's transference to manifest because of the fact that you will be relatively unknown to her and, yet, she will be plunged into a gloves-off environment with you.

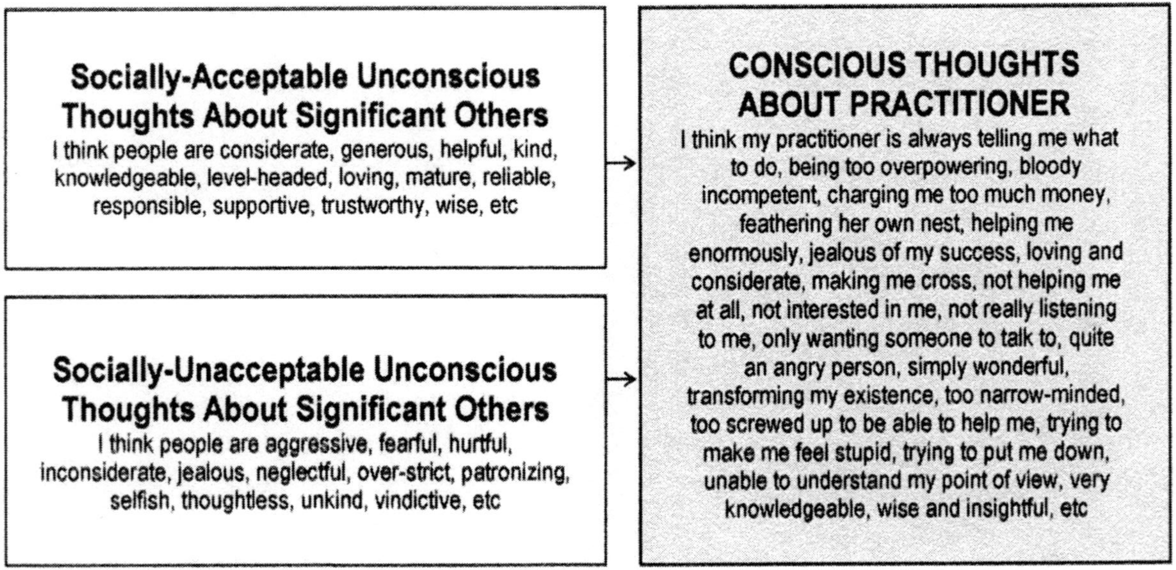

CONSCIOUS THOUGHTS ABOUT PRACTITIONER

I think my practitioner is always telling me what to do, being too overpowering, bloody incompetent, charging me too much money, feathering her own nest, helping me enormously, jealous of my success, loving and considerate, making me cross, not helping me at all, not interested in me, not really listening to me, only wanting someone to talk to, quite an angry person, simply wonderful, transforming my existence, too narrow-minded, too screwed up to be able to help me, trying to make me feel stupid, trying to put me down, unable to understand my point of view, very knowledgeable, wise and insightful, etc

Socially-Acceptable Unconscious Thoughts About Significant Others

I think people are considerate, generous, helpful, kind, knowledgeable, level-headed, loving, mature, reliable, responsible, supportive, trustworthy, wise, etc

Socially-Unacceptable Unconscious Thoughts About Significant Others

I think people are aggressive, fearful, hurtful, inconsiderate, jealous, neglectful, over-strict, patronizing, selfish, thoughtless, unkind, vindictive, etc

Figure 8.1 – *How might transference arise with your client?*

Cathartic transference will occur because it will be your client's primitive way of bringing unresolved matters to her mind's attention and, in doing so, she will be endeavoring to resolve these conflicts.

Therapeutic transference will arise in an unsuspecting and insidious manner for your client. Your client will travel through life with her unconscious thoughts, her opinions, her attitudes and her reactions to problem-people from long ago and will bring these into her current-day, closely-knit relationships. Your client will have been brought up in the social world and, consequently, she will have met people who were not always on her side. At best, your client's well-intentioned parents or her guardians were always telling her what to do and will have been dictating her choices. Your client may even have wished to rebel against these authority-figures who made her feel vulnerable and often inhibited her intended actions for fear of getting it wrong. At worst, life in your client's childhood will have been less than somewhat and she could have been neglected, rejected, abandoned, misused and/or abused by those responsible for her care and her upbringing.

The inestimable value of the therapeutic-transference phenomenon will be that your client's innermost thoughts and feelings about you may well arise mysteriously and, perhaps, be accompanied by a shock-reaction from the depths of her inner mind. The service that you will, undoubtedly, provide for your client, therefore, will be that she may have no other opportunity in her life for experiencing such insightful phenomenon outside your consulting room. Welcome your client's cathartic transference manifestation, in consequence, with open arms because you may, unwittingly, be doing her the biggest favor of her life and be assisting her healing process incomparably. Do not, however, fall into the trap of taking literally everything that your client says to you, or about you, to heart.

Ask yourself . . .

Has your client had her fair share of being misused by others? Was your client bullied at school and has she been pushed around at work? Do you suspect that your client will be unable to trust you or to have confidence in your sincerity? Could your client be far too frightened to let you into her personal space? Do you feel as if you are going into battle whenever you step into your consulting room with your client? Might your client appear to be developing an over-dependence on you and this situation rattles your cage somewhat? Do you feel really able to handle your client's transference manifestations and, if not, how does this make you feel? Would you consider that it could, now, be time for you to consult your supervisor because of the turbulent relationship that your client seems to have established with you? Do you take everything that your client says to you too literally? Can you detect and can you appreciate the behind-the-scenes significance of your client's cathartic transference manifestation?

How will you press your client's buttons?

The confidential therapeutic setting will be a particularly appropriate breeding-ground in which emotional baggage will surface for your client and, indeed, your treatment-strategy may well enhance this process. Moreover, if you are a relative stranger to your client, she will be more unconsciously inclined to project her problems and her issues on to you as her surrogate parent-guardian. Be assured that your client will recreate her own past in the guise of you as her unconsciously-chosen healing vehicle. In the therapeutic context, therefore, the climate will be ripe for fostering any unresolved transference and your client's projections will be magnified because of the supportive nature of your relationship with her, irrespective of your practice methodology.

Your client may, hopefully, regard you as her ideal carer and her reaction to you will take a positive and socially-acceptable shape. In this climate, therefore, you may make much headway with your client who can learn to trust you and to have confidence in your ability to supervise her healing program. On the other hand, your client may resist your therapeutic intervention when negative and socially-unacceptable transference reactions take hold of her and, for a while, you may find life an uphill struggle with her until she has resolved this factor. Your client, however, will learn an extremely valuable set of lessons about herself in facing and overcoming any negative transference towards you because she may make many important realizations about those significant others from her past from whom she felt unacceptable emotive distress.

When your client reacts to you in an incomprehensible way, therefore, you should regard this occurrence as a triumph. When the transference phenomenon manifests, in whatever form and in whatever circumstances, this will mean that you will be contributing, in some way, to your client's progress and you should be grateful for the privilege. Your best policy will be to appreciate this salient point and to allow your client's transference to take its course. Avoid the temptation, of course, to become personally offended when your client projects negative stuff on to you or, conversely, to preen your feathers when she worships the very ground on which you walk.

Ask yourself . . .

Does your client believe that you are somehow a superhuman being? Does your client show you the deference that she believes should be shown to the wise one? Does your client appear to be suspicious of your every move? Will your client show open hostility and overt rebellion towards you, despite the fact that you are earnestly attempting to help her? Does your client think you are a complete control-freak? Do you think your client has become infatuated with you just a tiny little bit? Does your client attempt to be over-friendly and very chatty with you when you really want to get down to work and your next customer is already in the waiting room? Are you able to simply trundle along and go with the flow in handling your client's reactions to you? Do you believe that your client will be judgmental about you and your work and will you take her opinions to heart? Does your client accuse you of failing her or of somehow mismanaging her treatment-program? Might your client appear to know more about you than you know about yourself? Does your client seem very self-opinionated and not backward in coming forward in stating her convictions? Can you sit on the fence when your client gives you her take on things? Can you allow your client's criticisms of you and your practice to simply slide off your back?

Let's take an example – Rosaline's story

Rosaline worked as a psychotherapist and part of her work routinely involved treating clients with relationship difficulties and with sexual dysfunction. It was part of Rosaline's normal practice to elicit information from any prospective client about any presenting problems before actually booking an appointment. On one occasion, a man rang to enquire about whether Rosaline was able to deal with his sexual dysfunction. Initially, this prospective client sounded genuine about seeking therapeutic assistance for his erectile dysfunction. Rosaline, of course, carefully explained what would be involved in psychotherapy and the way in which it could be of assistance to her prospective client.

Rosaline's potential client, nevertheless, seemed reticent about booking an appointment but was, also, reluctant to finish the telephone conversation and, so, she began to wonder why this was the case. Suddenly the man asked whether Rosaline would oblige him personally, in various ways, that would involve her in sexual activity with him. It seemed that this prospective client had truly failed to understand the scope and the limitations of psychotherapy. Rosaline blatantly refused this request but the enquirer protested that he was willing to pay extra. The only way of resolving this situation was for Rosaline to terminate the conversation with all due speed. This prospective client had, possibly, confused Rosaline with a former sexual partner or a lack of one.

How would you react to your client?

What will you discover about yourself from your relationship with your client? The way in which you might react to your client could take you unawares and be totally unpredictable in terms of the outcome for you.

Why will your client press your buttons?

Closely linked to the notion of transference will be the phenomenon of counter-transference whereby you will transfer your own particular issues on to your client (see Figure 8.2 – *How might counter-transference arise with you?*).

Your decision to become a therapeutic practitioner will usually be born out of the misfortunes of your own past experiences and this factor, then, will have, undoubtedly, prompted you to devote your life to a healing mission. You will need to recognize, somehow, the reasons why you chose to enter the caring profession as a means of compensating for what has happened to you

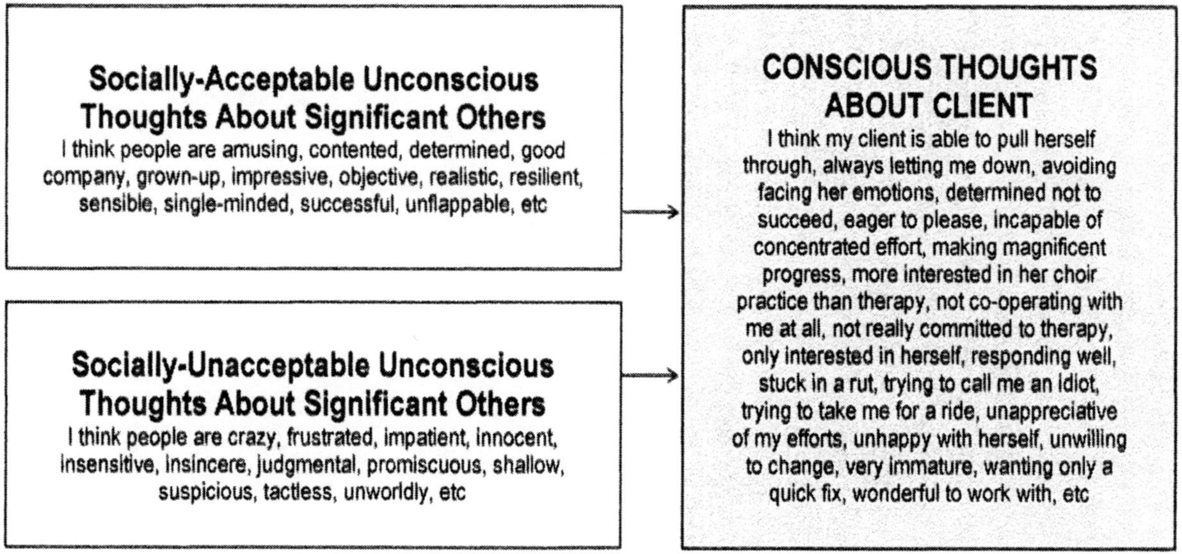

CONSCIOUS THOUGHTS ABOUT CLIENT

I think my client is able to pull herself through, always letting me down, avoiding facing her emotions, determined not to succeed, eager to please, incapable of concentrated effort, making magnificent progress, more interested in her choir practice than therapy, not co-operating with me at all, not really committed to therapy, only interested in herself, responding well, stuck in a rut, trying to call me an idiot, trying to take me for a ride, unappreciative of my efforts, unhappy with herself, unwilling to change, very immature, wanting only a quick fix, wonderful to work with, etc

Socially-Acceptable Unconscious Thoughts About Significant Others

I think people are amusing, contented, determined, good company, grown-up, impressive, objective, realistic, resilient, sensible, single-minded, successful, unflappable, etc

Socially-Unacceptable Unconscious Thoughts About Significant Others

I think people are crazy, frustrated, impatient, innocent, insensitive, insincere, judgmental, promiscuous, shallow, suspicious, tactless, unworldly, etc

Figure 8.2 – *How might counter-transference arise with you?*

in the past. If you had a reasonably supportive childhood, and are, now, continuing to further this care-taking interest, then, you may find yourself attracted to a therapeutic discipline that will offer similar scope in caring for and in nurturing others. If you had a pretty bumpy ride through childhood, however, you may well find yourself in a crisis-management profession that deals with big-time traumatic issues or with life-threatening diseases.

No individual can ever really survive childhood completely unscathed and, therefore, you will need to be a keen super-sleuth when your client has been making you react adversely as you might have done in the presence your own childhood guardians. When you feel at all uncomfortable or pushed off your perch by your client, then, take due note of your reactions. When the roller-coaster of your emotions takes an unexpected turn, allow this signal to be acknowledged. Your response to your client can, then, be traced back to its source in order to identify the originating cause of your unpredictable reaction. It may be quite understandable that your own unresolved, unconscious issues will be continually seeking an opportunity to get noticed and, so, fret not in these circumstances. This phenomenon will be in-evitable, at some stage, during your therapeutic career because no-one can ever actually escape this particular demon, although, now, you have been forewarned.

Possibly all the problems that you, as a practitioner, might encounter with your client could be whittled down to unresolved problems of counter-transference. If you feel sorrow over a perceived lack of love in your life, for instance, then, you may find that your client will appear indifferent to your plight and may seem to be only wrapped up in her own problems. If your self-confidence can easily be dented, then, you may find that your client will rob you, at the stroke of a pen, of any remaining vestiges of self-assurance. If you feel that you need to gain approval from others, then, you may wait, expectantly, for your client to say nice things about you. Examples of counter-transference could fill an entire volume alone but only you can identify your own particular concerns.

In all respects, counter-transference should be welcomed by you as a chance to gain further personal insight but, of course, the phenomenon should not be allowed to get out of hand with your client. You can usually learn to detect and to recognize the counter-transference phenomenon with your client in order to extinguish the demon before you say something to her that you might later regret. Failure to observe and to banish this gremlin may, of course, be detrimental both to your client and to your own peace of mind.

Often an index of your personal evolutionary progress will be to note that your client has, now, magically started to become supposedly better behaved. Your client, for instance, may not take advantage of your good nature too often or you will not feel obliged to bend the rules so readily for her sake. The more enlightened you become, of course, the more easily you will be able to attract the type of client who will give you maximum job-satisfaction every time without stirring up too much of your unresolved psychological baggage. If you do have significant difficulties with your client, then, you should, without delay, seek supervisory assistance. It may well be that most of the work that you will do with your supervisor will address your personal projection and your counter-transference issues. It could be said that counter-transference was the reason why supervision was invented in the first place because of the safe-haven that it can afford you.

Ask yourself . . .

Can you fully appreciate why you chose to enter the healing profession? Have you yet realized that you are practising as a healer in order to heal yourself? Are you a therapeutic practitioner because you have always known and always shown consideration for the wellbeing of others? Do you feel that you have a compulsive need to care for your client? Do you find that your client presses far too many of your psychological buttons? Does your client pull your guilt-strings quite regularly and does this take you by surprise? Can you learn to recognize and to work through your personal counter-transference issues with your client without beating yourself up? Do you fear that your client will make a complete fool of you and, then, will tell all her friends? Do you think that your client has been taking advantage of your good nature? Would you like your client to understanding things more from your point of view? Does your client rob you of your personal power and make you feel helpless and unruly? Can you strike a balance between having a sincere concern for your client and yet still run your life without her constantly being in your thoughts? Are you reminded of your own disease pattern when you are treating your client? Can you endeavor to take note of what your client might be telling you about your own ill-health or your chronic disorder? Do you believe that your opinion of your client does not get in the way of your therapeutic work? Do you feel that your counter-transference manifestation will affect your client, in some way, and that, maybe, it could be time for you to visit your supervisor?

Let's take an example – Charmian's story

Charmian works as a chiropractor and, in the course of her work, she deals regularly with clients who suffer from extreme stress and trauma. Somewhat mysteriously, Charmian found that she would receive a crop of clients who all seemed to be suffering from the same disorders or raising issues of a similar nature. For instance, for several weeks Charmian attended a number of clients who were suffering from grief issues or were exhibiting lower-back pain with some accompanying emotional distress. Charmian, initially, put these events down to coincidence but she soon found herself pondering on those issues that her clients had repeatedly raised.

Charmian decided to seek some personal supervision for topics that seemed to resonate most strongly with her in the course of her practice. From Charmian's own self-investigation, she soon discovered that her clients were reflecting many issues that had remained unresolved within her. Therefore, when Charmian was ripe for addressing her own unresolved grief, she found, as if by magic, that a number of her clients held underlying grief problems. Similarly, when emotional pain, that was connected with her lower back, was bubbling up to the surface, again, Charmian found herself noticing those specific issues that were exhibited by her clients. Other disorders from which her clients suffered, of course, passed relatively unnoticed because Charmian's buttons were not being insidiously pressed in these cases.

With monotonous regularity, therefore, Charmian began to notice that certain clients were acting as a very useful mirror in terms of what *she herself had next on the agenda to address. Once Charmian cottoned on to this phenomenon, those clients who were pressing her buttons began to perform a very useful role in assisting her with her evolutionary development by, unwittingly, resolving her inner conflicts and her personal malaise. Charmian, thus, was able to allow her clients to tell her what she needed to know about herself without her drawing any unnecessary conclusions about the suffering of others. By this means, Charmian was able to embrace counter-transference without letting it affect her work significantly.*

How will your client press your buttons?

Your client will press your buttons but you may only realize it after you have reacted dramatically. Your biggest demon may, indeed, arrive when your reaction to your client overspills into your consulting room. Always think out, in advance, what your plan of action will be in a catastrophic situation with your client. If you suspect that you are likely to become panic-stricken in front of your client, for example, then, seek help in order to guard against this occurrence. If you dread that you might burst into tears in your client's presence, then, be sure to have a stock set of phases that you could pull out in order to explain your reaction. If you fear that you may get a bit shirty with your client, then, ensure that you can stay tranquil, or wait until you have calmed down, before you open your mouth.

Working through inhibiting problems with your supervisor will give you sound peace of mind and will allow you to be impartial with your client. This course of action will enhance your life and, therefore, your client's care and wellbeing will automatically benefit. Remember that you are not infallible but should, in the therapeutic context, take responsible steps in order to protect your client. You can only do your best and not beat yourself up if things do go awry, although you should endeavor to deal responsibly with any disaster if it should strike.

You may, of course, need to cease providing therapy for any client who may be causing you interminable distress. You may wish to resort to drawing up some guidelines about whom you can and cannot treat, as a means of protecting yourself, until such time as you feel confident enough to handle any taxing cases. Do not ever put yourself in the direct firing line with your client if you can avoid this situation at all. Once you have resolved a given issue, then, you will be able to face the music without flinching in the future with your client. Riding the inevitable wave of reacting to your client and, then, undertaking the appropriate self-investigation will be your passport to widening the scope of your practice in terms of which cases you can actually tackle. This self-insightful process will be the very stuff of supervision and will ensure your successful survival as a dynamic practitioner.

The therapeutic interaction between you and your client will be like no other and, therefore, will be outside the realms of your everyday experience. For this reason, it may be a good idea for you to regularly stand back and to realistically view your relationship with your client. You could begin by considering the way in which you regard yourself as a communicator and an observer of mankind. You could, next, examine your interface with your client in the context of the unique therapeutic relationship that will have been formed with her and will, subsequently, develop during the course of her healing journey. Your ability to take a long, hard look at yourself will, no doubt, allow you to become a true and a confident healer with your client.

Ask yourself . . .

Do you get offended or feel like a failure when your client seems dissatisfied with what you have to offer her and she expresses her views openly? Could you feel responsible for your client's attitudes or her actions? Do you consider that your client has the power to bully you or to intimidate you? Will you endeavor to remain neutral yet find yourself taking sides when your client reports a confrontation with someone else? Might you feel obliged to pander to the whims of your client? Do you feel yourself spiraling out of control and powerless to avert disaster before it occurs? Do you consider that your client could be one of your dearest friends? Will you feel an overwhelming regard or an admiration for your client? Do you find that your client can make you feel insignificant, appear inefficient or feel despondent? Do you feel jealous of your client's financial position or her worldly success? Can you regard supervision as the safe-haven for you and your passport to self-enlightenment? Can you value your own reactions as a means of gaining better self-understanding and of becoming a more effective practitioner? Do you appreciate that you could, possibly, handle more taxing cases if you were to overcome your lurking doubts and your insidious fears? Does your difficult client leave you with a headache or cause you insomnia? Can you lose your appetite when you have had a bad day in the consulting room? Do you tend to become side-tracked by what your client says or what she does and this, then, prevents you from getting on with the job in hand? Might you catch yourself lowering your standards and giving second-best treatment to your client when the going gets tough? Do you find yourself having a long, chatty conversation with your client rather than administering your therapy?

Let's take an example – Adriana's story

Adriana is a reiki healer who, also, practices reflexology. At one point in Adriana's career, she began to feel exhausted and totally overwhelmed with life in general. Adriana, then, began to believe that she was soaking up the unwanted baggage of her client and this feeling took on a life of its own. When undertaking reiki healing, for example, Adriana could actually feel the physical and the emotional pain that her client was experiencing. Adriana, also, found herself shedding tears after a session when her client had related a tale of woe, despite her being merely an observer of the situation.

When Adriana's client talked about being heartbroken and/or feeling physical pain, she herself would experience this cardiac pain, together with some tightness in her chest on the following day. At the next session, however, Adriana's client reported that her pain had ceased but this was not much consolation to Adriana. Adriana felt that, on those occasions when she became susceptible to such reflected feelings, she was virtually unable to endure the exhaustion in the days that immediately followed seeing her client. In fact, Adriana's feelings were often so unbearable that she began to question her calling and to wonder why she had attracted certain clients. Adriana was, in addition, concerned about what she might, inadvertently, be sending back to her client.

It soon began to dawn on Adriana, however, that what she had ingested was more related to her own problems than to those of her client. One night, Adriana dreamed that she had assisted a woman in giving birth. In this dream, Adriana had disposed of the newborn baby, together with the afterbirth, but was, then, puzzled by her error. Adriana had, also, forgotten to cut the umbilical cord when the baby was born. Adriana, later, concluded that she was hounded by her ability to absorb stuff from her client and that her dream was showing her that she was unable to break free. With time, however, Adriana's feelings began to subside and she found herself less susceptible to the reactions of her clients. Adriana, thus, learned how to go with the flow of her own reactions and how to allot herself time and space when she needed it in order to deal with her own outpouring of emotional and physical infirmity. Adriana acknowledged that this was her body's way of jettisoning the malaise of her own past and, so, she soon acquired the skill of treating her client while simultaneously protecting herself.

How would you discover your own inner healer?

What will you discover about yourself when working with your client therapeutically? Becoming a practitioner will often entail looking at your own psyche in order to overcome your innermost doubts and fears about working as a professional. It may, in most circumstances, not be what your client does or what she says but your unique reaction to her that will be the most important factor in the overall equation.

How will you investigate yourself?

Often any self-torture that may beset you as a practitioner can be short-circuited by recognizing the phenomena of self-projection arising from within yourself and accepting it with equanimity as your inner wisdom (see Figure 8.3 – *How might self-projection arise with you?*).

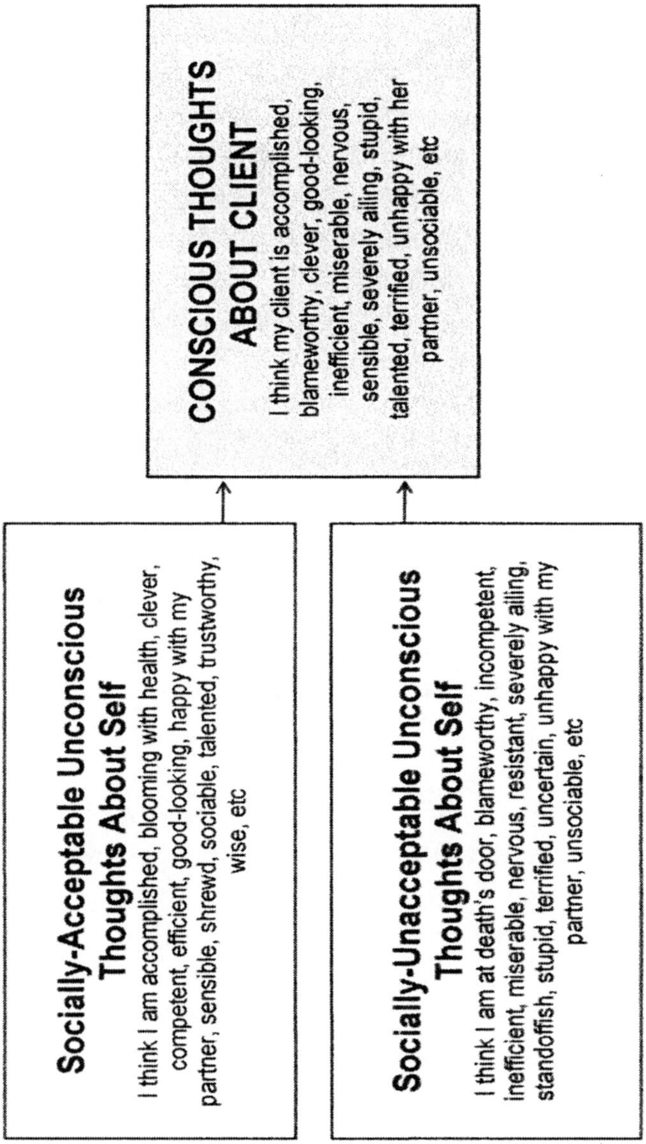

Socially-Acceptable Unconscious Thoughts About Self

I think I am accomplished, blooming with health, clever, competent, efficient, good-looking, happy with my partner, sensible, shrewd, sociable, talented, trustworthy, wise, etc

Socially-Unacceptable Unconscious Thoughts About Self

I think I am at death's door, blameworthy, incompetent, inefficient, miserable, nervous, resistant, severely ailing, standoffish, stupid, terrified, uncertain, unhappy with my partner, unsociable, etc

CONSCIOUS THOUGHTS ABOUT CLIENT

I think my client is accomplished, blameworthy, clever, good-looking, inefficient, miserable, nervous, sensible, severely ailing, stupid, talented, terrified, unhappy with her partner, unsociable, etc

Figure 8.3 – *How might self-projection arise with you?*

When you make a judgment about your client or you adopt an attitude towards her and, yet, you have very little evidence on which to support your thought-process, you may wish to consider whether you are projecting any aspects of your own psyche, or your own symptomology, on to her. In an intimate setting, such as will be afforded in the therapeutic environment, you may find yourself unconsciously imagining characteristics or may envisage conditions that your client may or may not actually exhibit. You can only see the world through your own eyes and, therefore, you could be tempted to perceive that your client thinks, feels, acts and tackles life in the same way as you do. If you make this brave assumption about your client, however, you are very likely to be wrong.

You may think good and praiseworthy things about your client or, conversely, you may not be so generous in your criticism. You may think, for instance, that your client should be undertaking your therapy in a certain way because that route has worked for you in the past. You may think that your client appears sorrowful or seems grief-stricken because you are harboring this underlying feeling. You may believe that your client might be ambitious and successful because you wish to be so, and could be positively moving in that direction, yet you do not really wish to acknowledge this fact overtly.

You may believe that your client has developed, or has been suffering from, a given disease or a particular malfunction because her symptoms match those of your own. You may believe that your client should be treated for a certain disorder because you have been afflicted in that way in the past. You may imagine that your client would dread to plunge into the depths of her innermost turmoil because you recall your own reluctance to venture into this terrain. You may sincerely believe that your client has been affected by a given set of circumstances, or a specific disease profile, when, in reality, she has experienced what she considers to be far more devastating tragedies.

When what your client might report seems to resonate distinctly with your own particular circumstances, however, she may be merely bringing you the gift of enlightenment. What you have noticed will be important for you just because you have noticed it. Life can have an uncanny way of showing you what you already know about yourself but might still need to hear from an independent source. The secret formula will be for you to recognize your self-projection as a product of your own experience and your self-concept and, subsequently, to resolve it as a favor to yourself. When you have recognized that you are projecting your stuff on to your client, however, do not, then, indulge in self-flagellation. Simply sit down, analyze your issue and work through this particular little demon, perhaps, if necessary, with the aid of a supervisor or with the help of a peer practitioner. In undertaking self-exploration, you will learn to protect yourself and not to prostrate yourself in order to please or to appease your client. The route towards capturing your personal demons will be self-observation and self-investigation in order to progress and to evolve as a dynamic therapeutic practitioner. By this means, you will uncover insights about yourself and, simultaneously, will become better acquainted with your healer within.

Ask yourself . . .

Will treating your client be an effortless task or a difficult operation? Does your imagination run away with you when you are treating your client? Does your client appear to have opinions about herself that differ from your own assessment of the facts about her? When your client looks happy, can you recognize that same joy within yourself? When your client appears pessimistic about the future, can you check to see whether this might not, in fact, be your own belief? Are you convinced that your client has contracted some form of serious killer-disease? If you are at death's door, do you believe that your client should be booking the undertaker just in case? When your client fails to make progress, do you recall the struggles that you might have had with your own healing journey? Do you think that your client has not been making progress and, yet, she appears to be perfectly content with her achievements to date?

Would you expect yourself to be a miracle-worker?

Will you put yourself up on a pedestal when working with your client? As a dedicated professional, you may constantly judge yourself by your client's attitude, her performance and her rate of recovery. This may be your way of expecting the impossible of yourself. It will, of course, be sheer and utter folly to judge yourself in terms of what your client might be able to achieve. Your client's success or her failure will be what she alone can attain. Perhaps the only way of evaluating your own success will be if you can claim that you enjoy your work.

How will you judge yourself?

If any progress your client makes might be greeted by you as an indication of your outstanding skill and competence as a therapeutic practitioner, you will, almost certainly, be making a cane for your own wrist. Think ahead to what will happen on those occasions when your client fails to make the grade. It might also be that by trying to be a magician, you will be putting some subtle pressure on your client to succeed and, right now, she could, possibly, do without any additional strain. It could, therefore, be said that you will be letting your client down by expecting yourself to be a miracle-worker and, thus, absolving her of taking any personal responsibility for her own health.

Do not take to heart your client's view of what therapy might be all about. Always remember that your client will be doing her recovery work in spite of your therapeutic expertise. Realize that it will be your client alone who must undergo her own healing crises. Never forget that you cannot directly influence the outcome of your client's therapeutic healing. Firmly hold on to the knowledge that you are merely a vehicle for and a facilitator of your client's recovery process. You do not need to over-identify with your client nor should you assume that you are, in any way, to blame for the machinations of her inner motivations. Self-blame will be an unproductive emotion and self-punishment will be a sheer waste of your precious time and energy and, certainly, will be of no use to your client. Your client should be quite able to take her own decisions in life and should, of course, be permitted to do so freely.

Your client's reaction to her therapeutic route will be her own personal contribution to the process and cannot be influenced by you, in any significant way, whatsoever. Even in exceptional cases of professional misconduct, your client will, still, have had a choice to get out of her sticky dilemma, to report the incident and to retaliate somehow in her own defence. Any failure in this respect, therefore, may be an important lesson for your client to have learned about herself and her boundary issues.

Let's look at it another way – The chocolate shop

A sweet-shop owner decides to sell some luxurious Belgian chocolates to his customers. The shopkeeper imports the most delicious and most expensive products and, then, displays them prominently in his shop-window. Customers flock in to buy these luxuries. A man wants to flatter his girlfriend. A woman wants to treat herself and to indulge her sugar-craving. A business executive wants to butter up a prospective customer. The customers arrive in their droves in order to partake of this new and self-indulgent delight, at last, available down at the local sweetie-shop.

When a customer elects to buy a box of Belgian chocolates, this, then, will be his personal choice, regardless of how much external persuasion might have influenced his decision. If the man does not succeed in seducing his girlfriend, or discovers that she does not even like chocolate, and that, therefore, the expensive gift was a sheer waste of money, then, that will be his problem. If the woman feels sick after eating an entire box of chocolates, or feels guilty about the weight that she will gain, that, still, will be her problem. If the business executive does not manage to win the contract from his customer, that, too, will be his problem. No guarantee can ever be given that the purchaser's underlying motivation for buying the chocolates will be successful and nothing to this effect will ever be written on the box.

It will not be the concern of the shopkeeper to adjudicate whether someone would be advised to eat chocolate, at all, or to purchase his brand of chocolate for any given reason. The shopkeeper may attempt to advise, or even to persuade, his potential customer but the buyer alone will make his final decision. The shopkeeper will be there offering goods for sale but the customer will be the one who must make the choice and must take the opportunity to spend his money, if he so desires.

Let's take an example – Roderigo's story

Roderigo encountered some problems when starting out in practice as a hypnotherapist that stemmed from his lack of confidence about interacting with his clients. Roderigo was, particularly, anxious about any false accusations that might be lodged by any dissatisfied client as a result of his inexperience. During a therapy session, in the early days, therefore, Roderigo was acutely aware of himself as a novice and was frightened that he would get something wrong with his client. Roderigo feared that he would not know immediately how to deal with a given issue for his client or not know what questions to ask in order to get at her truth. Roderigo sought advice from his supervisor and this helped a great deal but, of course, any possible solutions would, then, arrive with the benefit of hindsight.

Roderigo coped with his fears by focusing on his unique abilities and his life experience and by trusting that the future would turn out as he would have wished it to be. Roderigo's doubts about his ability, however, diminished in time as he gained experience and he learned how to handle complex situations. To date, no-one has ever complained about Roderigo's methods and he, now, trusts that any such complaints will either not be forthcoming in the future or, if necessary, he will be able to mount an effective defence by simply telling the truth.

Sometimes Roderigo used the well-tried trick of asking the universe for more clients and they usually came at his request. Roderigo, also, found that any dearth of new clients would normally, very conveniently, coincide with times when he had other more pressing commitments. Moreover, when Roderigo was able to give sufficient time to his work, and had mustered the energy in order to promote his business, then, the phone began to ring. When Roderigo resorted to asking the universe for help, therefore, he was simultaneously always ready to receive it.

Would you expect yourself to be a perfectionist?

Will you or your client ever succeed in being perfect? Anyone who aspires to the lofty height of perfectionism will, by definition, always fail miserably. The bad news will be that the perfectionist-trap has to be a catch-22 situation. If you aim for utter perfection, of course, it will just not be worth the continually-expended effort.

How will perfectionism manifest for you?

Your role as a practitioner will be to facilitate your client's journey and not to impose exemplary therapy upon her from a magnificent height. Often when you start out on your mission to heal others, you may have a preconceived notion of the way in which you should operate. You may have had a doctrine instilled in you from training school about good practice. You may have taken a qualifying examination and been given an arbitrary grading that will dictate your opinion of your own performance. You may observe other practitioners in the field who will appear infinitely more skilled and talented. You may, of course, feel empowered by giving of your best and later sense disappointment if your level best might just not be good enough in your own eyes and, therefore, your confidence will plummet. Banish any such judgmental thoughts from your mind about your abilities in order to avoid playing the I-am-determined-to-hang-myself game.

Do not be over-anxious to succeed with your client, as this may convey itself to her as desperation on your part. Your client may, also, intuitively gain the impression that you do not have any confidence in her ability to make progress. Do not, moreover, fall into the trap of counting with pride all those times when your client gives you praise and you note her obvious delight. This stuff may be momentarily great for your ego but beware the iron fist in a velvet glove. Your very next client may utterly fail to appreciate your efforts and may even express her dissatisfaction with your service. Now what can you believe about your professional competence? If you believe your first client, you will be elated temporarily, only to be dashed down in despair by your uncharitable and ungrateful client who maligned you so unjustifiably. The safest option, as always, will be for you to steer the middle course and to give not a fig for the opinions of any client.

Often you can deem that any decision you might make about treating your client will have been the best that you could muster, at the time, and in the prevailing circumstances, but this may be all you can ever expect of yourself. Sometimes you will be lucky and will be able to hit the nail on the head with precision timing at the very second when it might be needed by your client.

This may, however, be a Utopia that you might never be fortunate enough to experience with your client. Until such a moment dawns, simply plod on and have faith that your client will eventually make the grade, in some respect, with or without your help. Remember always that your client should be using you merely as a vehicle in which to travel.

Should you, in fact, make a so-called error of judgment with your client, you will, of course, need to take some corrective action. There may be a number of ways of tackling a particular problem with your client and you may feel spoilt for choice in certain situations. The best way of approaching such a dilemma with your client would be to plunge in with confidence and to make any appropriate adjustments along the way. You can, of course, never be sure that you will have made the correct move but intransigence will not be helpful either to you or to your client.

Ask yourself . . .

How hard are you trying to be the perfect practitioner? Are you often far too over-anxious about your ability to succeed with your client? How frequently do you chastise yourself if you are not 100% accurate in your diagnosis and not completely successful in your treatment-strategy with your client? Do you believe that you can succeed with your client where others might have patently failed? Are you elated if your client pays you a compliment with regard to your handling of her treatment? Do you feel mortified when your client appears dissatisfied with your advice or with your remedy for her particular condition? Do you feel chagrined when your client appears to criticize you or to question your judgment? Are you putting unconscious pressure on your client to make an exemplary recovery in record time by trying to be too perfect yourself? Can you eliminate all "I must" and "I should" thinking from your vocabulary when practising your therapy? If you make an error of judgment, can you pick yourself up again and recover from the experience?

Let's take an example – Horatio's story

Horatio felt duty-bound to be a super-human practitioner when he first started in practice as a rebirthing therapist. Horatio had benefited tremendously from his training and from his personal therapy but, then, felt that he had a responsibility to help others to his maximum ability.

218

Horatio, however, was attempting to do the impossible by asking too much of himself and, in turn, he was expecting too much from his clients. Horatio, therefore, got caught in the trap of trying so hard to please his client, allowing her to outstay her welcome, not charging her enough money for her sessions and, of course, feeling utterly dejected if she did not appear to be progressing in a praiseworthy manner. What Horatio had intended to be a fulfilling career had, now, become a cross that he heavily bore and he, thus, became the victim of his own torture.

As time went by, Horatio naturally began to cool down in terms of his over-dedication to duty. Fortunately, Horatio managed to find a supervisor who was able to help him to work through his many dilemmas. It transpired that, as a child, Horatio had always been required to do the right thing in the eyes of his parents. Horatio had, consequently, grown up with the impression that he had to try just that little bit harder in order to succeed. Horatio's parents had, also, been in the caring profession themselves and he had witnessed his mother feeling obliged to become a doormat for others. This realization, together with the natural passage of time and his experience of working as a practitioner, brought a resolution to Horatio's obstacles.

Once Horatio began to emerge from the negative programming that he had received as a child, his personal boundaries began to strengthen. Horatio became more stringent with the time allocation for his sessions and the fees he charged. None of Horatio's clients was permitted to escape without paying, or given a reduced rate, because he had over-identified with them. Moreover, Horatio began to realize that it was his client's sole responsibility for recovery and that his work was only to help her further along the road. With more stringent boundaries in place, Horatio began to attract the type of client that he needed for success. Horatio, thereafter, found that his clients became more focused on getting well and, furthermore, were not an endless stream of quick-fix merchants and time-wasters. A successful hit-rate, now, meant that Horatio's practice expanded and this growth, subsequently, helped both his coffers and his degree of work-satisfaction.

How would you tell whether your work will be really effective?

Will you ever be able to prove that you have managed to get it right with your client? You may suffer endless torture in trying to measure your success with your client even though this may be an impossible task for you to accomplish.

What will you be trying to prove to yourself?

You cannot, in essence, ever measure or ever quantify whether you are, in fact, effective as a practitioner with your client. You cannot, therefore, truly judge, in any way, whether you have been successful as a practitioner. So relax and get used to this intriguing idea. Remember that your client cannot, in fact, reach the dizzy height of sheer perfection and, because a total cure may not be possible for her, all you are actually able to achieve, as a practitioner, will be to take her further along her healing road.

Success for your client will be totally relative in the entire equation of therapeutic practice. You may, for instance, be very pleased with the job you do with your client and, then, to your amazement, you will discover that she claims that she only feels slightly better. You may, conversely, consider yourself to be an utter failure with your client who, then, proudly announces that you have changed her life out of all recognition. Bear in mind that, under any circumstances, your client will still only be giving a subjective view of her recovery picture, or any lack of it, while you just remain an impartial observer.

Judgment of success, emanating either from you, or from your client, will be both relative and subjective value-judgments and, so, nothing could ever be proven definitively in this respect. The bottom line will be that no-one could ever prove in a court of law decisively, one way or the other, whether your client has made any significant progress at all towards recovery, whether she has merely freewheeled for a while or whether she has gone completely downhill. The best you can ever hope to claim might be that you will have made a difference, in some degree, with your client. Content yourself with this knowledge and relieve yourself of the burden of focusing on the outcome of your client's case as a means of self-evaluation.

Ask yourself . . .

Do you feel an obligation to your client to get it right every time? Perhaps your greatest enemy of all will be your attitude towards your own conduct with your client? Might you feel that all your client's woes are purely the result of attending your clinic? Do you worry if you have to make a diagnosis or a major decision about your client's condition? Will you dread that you could give the wrong advice, could suggest an inappropriate diet or might prescribe a useless remedy for your client? Do you consider that you might say something to which your client may take offence? Do you believe that you might be meddling with your client's mind or with her biochemistry? Would you feel unqualified to make a pronouncement about the state of your client's health? Do you worry that, if your client does not get better, she will tell all her friends and ruin your unblemished reputation?

Let's look at it another way – The life and times of the kestrel

The kestrel, Falco Tinnunculus, is a bird of prey commonly found throughout Europe, Scandinavia, Russia and North Africa. The kestrel will hover in flight 7 to 12 metres above the terrain when stalking his prey. When airborne, the kestrel will exercise his precision-tuned, binocular vision in order to detect his prey. The kestrel's quarry can be as gigantic as a hare or as miniscule as a worm. Once this majestic falcon has sighted his prey, he will, then, bide his time by encircling the territory and characteristically hovering expectantly. The kestrel, then, and only then, will have to make a decision. Will the kestrel decide to swoop, to remain hovering or to fly away in search of pastures anew?

If the kestrel spies a tasty meal, is feeling hungry and considers that he has enough energy in order to swoop, he will, undoubtedly, profitably secure his prize. If, however, the kestrel feels that he might not really be hungry, or that the atmospheric fluctuations are against him, he may wait until conditions are more favorable. Alternatively, the falcon may simply fly away and enjoy freedom in the breeze. The decision made by the kestrel, however, has nothing whatsoever to do with whether the leaves on the trees are green or gold, whether the sky is pure blue or overcast, whether the sun is shining, whether the wind is coming from the north, whether there is a light drizzle, whether some people are having a picnic or whether the moon is in Aquarius. The kes-

trel will make his own choices, and in his own time, because he will be as free as a bird to live his life as he pleases.

If the kestrel does decide to swoop on his prey, nonetheless, he may feel thoroughly satisfied by his meal and be pleased that he had toiled long and hard in order to secure his reward. The kestrel's own unique choice may have been based on need, on desperation or on a resolve to succeed. Atmospheric conditions may play some part in the falcon's decision-making process, perhaps, but, still, it will be his own personal choice alone.

If the kestrel elects to remain hovering in flight, then, he may have decided that, for his own reasons, the time might not be quite suitable just now. This does not mean that he will not seek another opportunity, in the future, to grasp that tasty nettle. This, also, does not mean that another object of prey will not present itself at a more appropriate time. The kestrel's decision does not mean that the trees were waving in the wrong direction or that the sun was not shining brilliantly enough.

If the kestrel decides to fly away and to seek another victim, or to go off to talk with his other feathered friends, he will do so. The kestrel may not be very hungry right now, that succulent morsel may not be enticing enough or he may just have other fish to fry. If the kestrel elects not to bother to capture his prey, at all, then, that will be his ultimate decision. If the kestrel elects not to pounce and to fly away, the sun will not indulge in self-blame, the wind will not change direction and those happy picnickers will still enjoy their smoked salmon and caviar. In which direction might you be flying?

Let's take an example – Imogen's story

Imogen, a craniosacral therapist, was dismayed to learn that her client planned to terminate her therapeutic sessions. Imogen had been treating her client for a number of disorders and some initial progress had, she felt, been made. Imogen's client announced, at her last session, that she had decided to seek counseling instead of craniosacral therapy for her insomnia because it was preventing her from returning to work. Imogen was taken aback by this news and felt that her client was leaving because she considered that craniosacral therapy could only deal with a body-focused condition. Imogen had, in fact, already incorporated verbal counseling skills into the treatment of her client and, therefore, she felt somewhat deserted and cheated.

Imogen began to feel inadequate and pondered on whether she should advertise the fact that she had learned some counseling skills from a pre-

vious course in spiritual psychotherapy. Moreover, Imogen was disturbed that her client had not realized that the greater includes the lesser in terms of holistic healing. Imogen, also, felt, conversely, that, perhaps, she did not have the right to utilize any verbal skills within her therapeutic discipline. Most of all, Imogen considered that she was not being taken seriously as a true professional and she, therefore, felt indignation at her client's flippant and closed-minded attitude to her own health.

This mishmash of conflicting thoughts plagued Imogen until she realized that her reaction was intense because of the attitude that her father had often taken to her knowledge and her intelligence in the past. Throughout her childhood and her adulthood, Imogen's father, for instance, would adopt the premise that she was too young and too innocent to know certain facts about the ways of the world. In fact, Imogen's relationship with her client, and her reaction to being supposedly deserted, had a direct parallel to the relationship she had formed with both her parents. This understanding, then, took the heat out of the situation for Imogen.

Imogen, also, realized that her client was actually after a quick-fix and that pressure had been brought to bear on her by her family who were expecting her to make a speedy recovery. Imogen, furthermore, began to appreciate that her treatment may well have touched her client in such a way that it would have stirred within her the realization that some in-depth therapy would be needed in order to pull herself out of the quagmire. With this new-found enlightenment, Imogen soon recognized that she was, in fact, probably better off without her former client.

How would your client be doing?

Will your client's perceived lack of progress be doing your head in? As a practitioner, the one overriding, albeit unnecessary, worry that you may harbor will be whether your client may, in fact, be getting any better at all and your greatest fear, of course, may be that she will not. Be prepared to let go of this particular demon with all due speed and just get used to living with this familiar degree of uncertainty.

Will your client be making any progress?

You may never be able to tell, let alone prove, whether your client will be capable of improving, or whether she will ever improve, her condition. Feel safe in the knowledge that you will be making some difference to your client, in some respect, merely by virtue of the fact that she will spend time in your company. Be assured, moreover, that your client could get better in spite of you. Your client's recovery or her health improvement, of course, may not have anything to do with you, at all, however hard you might have been trying.

Your client's progress may not be obvious especially from the perspective of an obsessed observer. You may, of course, not overtly notice your client's improvement and, possibly, the more you look, the more you will not see. Even your client may not be aware of any significant change and this situation will be the test of your stamina in terms of continuing to believe in yourself. Do not be tempted to brand yourself as an absolute failure and to get into any self-punishing mode just because your client might be dragging her coat.

You may be seeing your client over a continuous period of time and may not be able to see any overall change. Your client's major shifts, hence, may not be detectable to your naked eye. Furthermore, do not expect your client to have monumental insights, or to make a stupendous improvement, at every session. You may think that because you get hungry every day that it would be a good idea for you to eat a week's food at one meal and, then, save on the washing up for the rest of the week. In practice, of course, this could not happen and it would be laughable even to suggest this possibility. Why, then, would you put the same kind of pressure either on yourself or on your client by using such nonsensical logic?

The main point to emphasize here will be that if your client gets better magnificently, if she remains in the same aimless state or even if she declines rapidly, then, none of this will be your doing. As a practitioner, you will merely be the trolley-bus on which your client chooses to travel. By all means be a responsible and caring practitioner but do not take your client's concerns to heart. If you have extreme difficulty with this issue, then, resoundingly knock on the door of your supervisor and, additionally, undertake some mind-exploration around your tendency to self-blame or to over-identify with others.

Ask yourself . . .

Perhaps your client meets herself too regularly and, so, she will not notice any gradual change? Maybe your client has been following her usual recovery-pattern of being in denial about change? Perchance your client's health improvement may not readily be emerging because of her current healing crisis? Perhaps you have neglected to recognize that your client's health picture will, currently, be a complete matrix of her past but that this image is, at last, breaking up? When your client has a major remedial shift during or after your first session, will you, then, expect a mountain to be moved every time you see her in the future? Do you hang on your client's every word for evidence of her progress and her success? When your client may be undergoing a healing crisis, does she tend to think that it must be your fault? Have you explained clearly to your client what to expect from your therapeutic methodology and from any healing crises? Are you over-fond of blaming yourself for everything that goes wrong in the world? Did your parents or your guardians have a tendency to chastise you frequently as a child? Were your always regarded as the black sheep of your family?

Let's look at it another way – Flying a kite

It is a blustery day and quite perfect for flying a new kite. It is warm on the ground with a rising air-current and, yet, the tops of the trees are waving not too violently in the breeze. The skilled kite-flyer will assess the weather and, then, set out for a day of fun. The kite-flyer will skillfully launch his kite into the breeze after making an assessment of the direction of the wind and the climatic conditions. The kite-flyer will, perhaps, have had a number of tryouts before allowing the kite to soar into the skies. The kite-flyer may, also, have made some abortive attempts and, hence, given up on previous days because the weather conditions were unfavorable at that time.

Once the kite has been launched, the kite, itself, may be very visible but the kite-strings will be utterly invisible from a distance. Someone else, standing some distance away, may see the kite flying in the sky but not see the strings or even the kite-flyer himself. This observer may watch the kite dancing, dipping and diving at the mercy of the wind. The onlooker may, then, admire the skill of the kite-flyer without actually being able to see him. The observer, of course, will not be able to see the way in which the kite-flyer

225

has been pulling the strings and will be unaware of any previous failures to launch the kite. The spectator may, therefore, only perceive the kite-flyer's success and will generalize that he will invariably be unbeaten. What kind of a kite might you be flying?

9 WHERE WOULD YOU BE RIGHT NOW?

What would it be like being a practitioner?

Will you be on the inside looking out or on the outside look-ing in when healing your client? When you become a professional alternative practitioner, the world about you will, undoubtedly, change irrevocably and there will be no going back once the die has been cast. It may seem as if you are suddenly plunged into a parallel universe once you have started on that journey of self-discovery. You could travel the world but, then, realize that you will actually see more of the truth about human nature from the confines of your consulting room.

What will the world think about you?

The therapeutic profession might, possibly, be one of the most misunderstood of vocational occupations. Many practitio-ners even studiously avoid referring to their work as a result of the many preposterous misconceptions that the raw public will often retain about the role of the therapeutic practitioner. The average man in the street may give but a vague and embarrassed grin when you state that you are an alternative practitioner. The great unwashed may show childish fascination or, perhaps, even effusive enthusiasm when you casually mentioned your occupa-tion at a social gathering. The man in the street may make trite comments like "I bet you meet some really interesting people?", "Well, we all eat a lot of junk-food really!" or "I suppose you have psychoanalyzed me already?". Alternatively, the casual partygoer may politely excuse himself and swiftly find a proper mortal with whom he can safely converse.

The other side of the coin will be that, once at a gathering of the therapeutic clans, the conversation among fellow-practitioners will exhibit an excited fervor when all can be assured of the knowledge that others will be on the same wavelength and will not, therefore, react adversely or behave bizarrely.

Ask yourself . . .

Do you feel somewhat socially isolated by possessing personal knowledge that many others obviously do not? Might you wish, now, that you had not rubbed the magic lamp? Are you, nowadays, constantly amazed at the simplistic reactions and the primitive motivations of others? Do you, at last, feel as if people are suddenly utterly transparent? Has your healing journey set you apart even from those close to you? Are you appalled at the dangerous way in which the man in the street abuses his health? Do you feel that you have arrived in an exclusive club? Have you ever regretted your therapeutic journey or your introduction into the world of self-enlightenment?

What will you think about the world?

As a practitioner, your view of the world may change to such an extent that you will regard Mr Average as an unenlightened freak. When you have discovered your own destiny, you may find that those who do not jump on the bandwagon with you could appear to be very much out-of-step, as if newly arrived from another planet. Personal enlightenment and personal freedom from ill-health may often be a hard legacy for you to inherent and it may surprise you when you find yourself landed with it. Your new-found insight may be a disturbing phenomenon to which you will need to adjust. Your key to good health, however, may be one that you cannot automatically hand to others. You may not require counseling in order to live with the shock but you will need to overcome the strangeness and to accept this phenomenon as the norm in your life from this moment onward.

Life as a therapeutic practitioner has often been regarded as a lonely road but it should, also, be viewed as an evolutionary journey for you as an individual in your own right. Frequently, your mission will require that you come to terms with those inner feelings of being different or even superior to others. Acknowledge that such reactions may be a vital part of your healing path and that eventually the territory will not seem so strange and that soon you will be able to accept others with equanimity. A feeling of somehow being different from others, and not accepting this fact with level-headedness, could, of course, tempt you to go over the top in terms of being a healer. Worry not if this happens. Simply tell yourself that this will be a necessary element of your healing experience and that this phase will soon pass, although do remain vaguely aware of what could be happening to you.

Ask yourself . . .

Do you find yourself estranged from others because of your newly-acquired therapeutic enlightenment? Do you wonder from whence your psychic ability has magically sprung? Are you amazed when some people continually whinge, gossip and complain? Are you puzzled when others continue to protest that they are utterly invincible and supremely faultless? Will you be astounded because a certain man endlessly gets himself into a scrape from which he cannot seem to dig himself out? Do you question why a certain woman persists in putting up with the stick from others? Do you understand why a despairing man does not realize that there could be another way? Are you concerned because an unhappy woman feels that everything must, somehow, be her fault? Do you want to urge a despondent man to get off his arse and just get on with it? Do you wonder why a worried woman needs to feel anxious every hour of the day? Can you see most people's problems, now, as being crystal clear? Can you actually appreciate where a close friend might be coming from? Do you wonder why the world still continues to suffer unnecessarily from arthritis, from migraines, from heart disease and from stomach upsets?

Let's take an example – Nerissa's story

Nerissa set up in practice as a spiritual psychotherapist and psychic healer. Nerissa gave up her daytime job in order to focus on her new career because she wished to be self-employed and to be financially independent. Nerissa found that, because of her extensive experience of therapeutic practice from the lying-on-the-couch angle, she could very much understand where her client was coming from. Moreover, Nerissa had developed a degree of freedom and openness that she found conveyed itself naturally to her client. Nerissa could, therefore, be herself in her own consulting room, could feel confident in her work and could be honest with herself and with her client. With these qualities in tow, Nerissa had little difficulty in attracting clients once she had started to build up her practice and when she had begun to obtain referrals from previous clients.

For Nerissa, therefore, the expansion of her business was a natural progression from being a client herself to opening up an area of her life that became personally and financially rewarding because she simply enjoyed what she did. Nerissa, also, found that her practice expanded because of the high number of referrals that she regularly received and, when this occurred, her financial outlay on advertising, correspondingly, decreased. In Nerissa's case, therefore, success bred additional income and this upward trend resulted merely from self-belief and from taking pleasure in her work as a natural form of self-evolution.

Where would you be coming from?

What will you see when you look back on your life and your work with your client? You might wish to seriously consider the way in which your personal development has dovetailed into the holistic framework. When viewing yourself as a practitioner, it will be important for you to get yourself into your own unique perspective. You will, then, be able to see yourself in terms of your personal evolution and your particular ability to gain job-satisfaction.

When will you have first become a practitioner?

The point at which the practitioner within you will have decided to emerge will usually be dictated by your life circumstances or, possibly, triggered by some necessity. Your turning point will normally be vividly remembered, although its inception may be obscured from your overt consciousness. Any or all of the reasons why you became a practitioner, in the first place, will contribute to the way in which you approach your work and the way in which you will personally evolve. Spend some time, therefore, in solemnly examining yourself and your personal motivations as these will be the key to your entwined personal and professional development.

Ask yourself . . .

When did you first feel the conviction to help others in a beneficial way? Do you feel the need to make a positive contribution to this world in order to relieve some of the suffering of others? Do you feel privileged to have learned ways in which you can prolong your life and those of others? Did your turning-point in life occur when you felt thoroughly disillusioned by the façade of the unreal world? Could your existence have utterly changed when you started to rebel against social pretences, entrenched dogma, cultural pressures and the high-tech approaches to medicine? Did you get a wakeup call when your health failed, your emotional state took a nosedive and your life utterly fell apart at the seams? Did your moment of enlightenment arrive when you wanted to break free of the vice-like grip of towing the line and being normal? Might you have had a moment of illumination when you realized that there must be more to life than earning a crust in the interminable rat-race? Did sheer frustration with your own inability to make things work productively bring you to a point of realization? Did you have a flash of inspiration when you realized that you could help yourself and simultaneously assist others?

Let's take an example – Gregory's story

Gregory had been close to someone who was in great emotional pain but, at that time, his partner was offered only heavy doses of drugs as treatment. Gregory felt, instinctively, that there must be a better way and, thus, began his search for a satisfactory resolution in order to assist his partner.

Gregory decided to become a reiki practitioner while still working full-time and this practice set him on his healing path. Gregory found, however, that his reiki treatment would bring about emotional reactions in his client but he, still, considered that there was no way in which he could actually help her to overcome her painful responses. Gregory, hence, had gained some fulfillment from his work but he, also, felt sure that he wanted to take it further towards a more satisfactory conclusion for his client.

In his search, Gregory discovered hypnotherapy when it helped him personally during his crisis with his partner. Gregory's personal experience with in-depth analytical hypnotherapy demonstrated to him that it would be possible for him to offer hope to people who suffer in adult-

hood as a result of childhood experiences. With this discovery, Gregory, hence, decided that he wanted to follow a profession in which he could decisively help others. Gregory believed that his clients could be given an opportunity to avoid some of the tragedies that he had, himself, suffered throughout his life. When Gregory had been made redundant from his job for the second time, therefore, he saw and he seized an opportunity for self-employment by setting up in practice as a hypnotherapist.

How would you reflect on your therapeutic journey?

Will you need to closely examine your personal healing journey under the microscope when working with your client? Becoming a practitioner will be a strange metamorphosis for you. It could be rather like going through a tunnel without any light at the end, without any illumination on the way, without any official guide and without any conscious reason for your journey.

When will your therapeutic evolution have begun?

Endeavor to reflect on your therapeutic journey in order to appreciate its significance and its impact on your life's purpose. This self-examination will put your work as a healer into the appropriate perspective. Allow yourself to ponder on the past in order to identify when you first set out on your journey with the aim of becoming a therapeutic practitioner. Observe, too, the path that you have taken in order to bring your aspirations to fruition.

Consider your therapeutic journey to date and visualize that moment in time when it all started for you. You may instantly think that your therapeutic journey began on the very first day of your initial training course but often this observation will not be quite truly accurate. Nearly always, as a practitioner, you will have been born to the profession or, at least, it may seem that way. Therapeutic work will not normally be something that will be advocated by your careers teacher at school. You are unlikely to have chosen to become a healing practitioner because you could not make up your mind about what you wanted to do when you grew up. You may not have seen an advertisement for the profession down at the local job-center.

Becoming a practitioner will usually occur in your more mature years, of course, when life experience has taken its toll. Your life will tell its own story and, in reflecting on your life, you will usually see the pattern emerging quite distinctly. This self-observation exercise will let you know truly where you are coming from. From this vantage point, you will, then, be able to see the path ahead more clearly and will be able to fulfill your potential both as a therapeutic practitioner and as an individual.

Ask yourself . . .

In what ways does your life experience reflect your role as a therapeutic practitioner? Can you remember caring for others at school or for your parents at home? Can you recall being consulted by friends and by acquaintances as the wisest sage? Do you see glimpses of the healer within you emerging in your previous occupation? Perhaps you were required to make a few mistakes along the way before launching yourself into the role of assisting others who have made similar errors? Maybe you will have needed to sow some wild oats before settling down into your chosen profession? Maybe your therapeutic work has echoed from the past for many years? Can you recall looking after your parents, your guardians or your siblings when you were only a child yourself?

How will you reflect on the road you have taken?

Allow yourself to consider your therapeutic journey in the context of your life's comprehensive picture. Meditate on the way in which you have arrived at this point in time in your life. Pinpoint the moment, in your past, when you discovered your gifts and, then, trace the way in which these attributes have unfolded for you.

Begin by picturing the moment when you were born into this world. Imagine who was there and how those present reacted to your arrival. Now consider every step along the way towards becoming a practitioner. Note every occasion when you assisted someone else or when you wanted desperately to do so. Record every knock and every scrape that set you up for experiencing life in the raw. Recall any personal hardship that gave you the tools to assist others. Examine, piece by piece, those events in your life that shaped you and molded you for a career in the therapeutic profession.

Pinpoint the precise moment in time long ago when you, first, decided to become a helper of others. Discovering this pearl in the oyster may not be straightforward initially but, with due reflection, the picture will emerge from the depths of your innermost voice. Now trace your path from the moment of the inception of your chosen journey to the point when you finally decided to take the plunge into alternative practice. Map out every decision that you took and every corner that you turned along the way towards your goal. Observe the hills and the valleys along the winding road, the laughs, the tears, the sunshine and the showers. Visualize yourself developing and emerging from a casual helper into a fully-fledged therapeutic professional.

Clearly recall the moment when you saw your first practice-client while you were still in training. Recall, too, your trepidation, excitement, uncertainty, confusion, elation and uneasiness when dealing with your very first fee-paying client. Take stock of where you are now. See the route that you have taken in order to arrive in your current position. Watch the progress that you have made as if you were unfolding a flower at dawn. Observe the good times and the not-so-good times and discover what you have learned from the many trip-ups along the way. But note that progress has, in some way, been accomplished by you personally and know, in your own heart, that advancement will inevitably continue in a similar vein because that will be the way of the world.

Speculate, for a moment, now, on what the future might hold for you based on your previous evolutionary history. The wave that begins far out at sea will, without fail, eventually reach the shore and will tickle your toes. Stay faithful to this memory of the past as your means of creating your own future.

Ask yourself . . .

What has your reflection on your own personal, therapeutic journey thrown up for you? Can you appreciate that you saw your very first client long before you actually began to practice as a paid professional? Can you regard yourself as a fully-fledged practitioner from the moment of treating your first practice-client on your initial training course? Did you feel elated at your success, or chagrined by any perceived blunders that you might have made, when you saw your first client? When you treated your first client, did you feel spurred on to greater things or, conversely, reticent about meeting your next customer? When you initially gave someone a treatment, did you feel that you possessed the necessary attributes for victory in the field or did you consider giving up and returning to the drawing board? As you saw your first client, did you feel a composite of many mixed emotions and blinding thoughts? Can you see, now, how your past can create your personal future? Do you still believe that you have made little or no progress as a practitioner?

Let's take an example – Malvolio's story

Malvolio decided to train as an osteopath after a period of indecision about his future career. Malvolio enjoyed his training because it gave him purpose, provided him with a direction to his life and gave him much hope for his future. Malvolio wanted to take up a career that would give meaning to his life and would help him to come to terms with the tragic loss of his father who had died suddenly.

The duration of Malvolio's training took 5 years and he learned much about himself in that time. Notwithstanding the fact that 5 years will be a significant chunk of anyone's life, Malvolio had not bargained for the dramatic personal change that he would undergo during this extensive period of time. Malvolio, thence, emerged from his training experience as a completely different person. Malvolio's outlook on life, his ideals, his values and his thinking had all been transformed and he emerged from this morass with a new psychological mindset.

Once Malvolio's illusions about himself and his life had been shattered by his therapeutic training and his journey of self-discovery, the inevitable result was a major life-change for him. The final outcome was that Malvolio separated from his partner and his children and this event was accompanied by all the upheaval and the drama that such a break-up will inevitable entail. But for Malvolio there was no going back because he could simply not put the jack back into the box.

Why would you have become a practitioner?

Will you know why you have a caring practitioner's blood in your veins when treating your client? Your health evolution and your own therapeutic journey will, in most cases, dictate the nature of the therapy, or the therapies, that you will practice. Your reason for taking up the practitioner's reigns, therefore, will be an important factor in the overall equation.

Why will the bell have tolled for you?

Your own positive experience will, in most cases, become your passport to spreading the word on the been-there-and-got-the-teeshirt basis. Any successful form of self-enlightenment and any personal recovery from ill-health will prescribe your outlook on the therapeutic domain and will dictate your whole concept of the healing process. You may, now, practice what you preach, tread the well-trodden path and live your own personal truth.

It may be important for your self-confidence for you to realize that the person you are, currently, and the person you have been, in the past, will be your greatest asset and may constitute a vital ingredient in your therapeutic equation. You may, for instance, be someone with experience of world travel, high finance and/or being in the media spotlight and, hence, your client may be attracted by these accomplishments. You may have some special knowledge of a given industry or a certain profession that will assist you in running your business. You may come to your specific therapeutic profession after a career in another caring field, such as teaching, nursing or pharmacy, that will throw a unique light on your alternative practice. You may be a parent, who will be well versed in the trials and tribulations of parenthood, and this experience will assist you when handling clients of all ages and at all stages in life. All the ingredients that you put into the mixing bowl will affect the taste of the final pudding.

Your personal experience of life, and the ways in which you have overcome any distress, will, of course, make you the person you are and the practitioner you will continue to become. Your personal experience of childhood distress, chronic illness, drug-taking, enterprise success, financial hardship, physical injury, unemployment, unsuccessful relationships and wild-parties, for example, will all, paradoxically, assist you as a practitioner throughout your career. The man in the street, of course, would normally be astounded by this pearl of wisdom.

Your own healing journey may continue with further and regular personal therapy, a thoroughly praiseworthy diet and an exemplary lifestyle, if you so desire. Your therapeutic enlightenment may, now, mean that your interest in the spiritual health of the planet, the nutrition of the nation, the prospects for the environment and your own personal ecology system will be a good advertisement for healthy living in its entirety. The ideals of therapeutic doctrine may be great for you but, of course, it may be the parting of the ways for others who do not wish to adopt your regime.

Ask yourself . . .

Did you become a practitioner for a whole multiplicity of complex and inter-related reasons? In what ways does your therapeutic discipline reflect your personal experience of success in therapy? Did you save your own life by expelling the toxins or by correcting a serious biochemical deficiency? Might you have overcome a life-threatening disease through alternative thinking? Did you claw your way back from the jaws of suicidal depression or from monstrous anxieties? Would you once have suffered from panic attacks, from agoraphobia or from a severe lack of confidence? Would you have gained enlightenment, received a life-affirming calling or investigated the deeply spiritual realm as a result of an unhappy experience or any extreme ill-health? Did you suddenly realize that you could flourish on a diet of healthy living? Have you regained physical functionality or bodily mobility and have you achieved your ultimate aim of freedom from agonizing pain? Are you any longer crippled by your own health deterioration? Did you overcome a life-threatening condition in a way that others have not been able to? What kind of working career did you follow prior to becoming a practitioner? In what ways can you capitalize on your previous working experience when practising as a therapist?

Let's take an example – Virgilia's story

Virgilia began taking flower essences after the premature and unexpected death of her father when she was a young adult. At this time in her life, Virgilia had been put on anti-depressants by her general medical practitioner because she had been unable to cope with the shock of her bereavement. Moreover, Virgilia had been obliged to look after her widowed mother. Once Virgilia had begun to experiment with flower essences, she soon began to recover from her bereavement issues. Simultaneously, this healing stimulated Virgilia's interest in the whole subject of Bach flower essences and Australian bush flower essences about which she read avidly and, subsequently, signed up for a practitioner's training course.

Later in life, Virgilia found herself struggling with an intensely painful and isolating experience – that of having difficulty with conceiving a child and of undergoing a number of distressing miscarriages. Virgilia, then, tried many different therapies, such as acupuncture, reflexology, homeopathy and nutritional therapy, but she still remained childless. Following one of her miscarriages, Virgilia found out about a diploma in vibrational medicine and it transpired that she had all the right entry qualifications in order to sign up. Two years later, Virgilia had become qualified and was, then, the proud owner of over 20 ranges of flower essences. During her two-year training course, Virgilia, also, engaged in psychotherapy with a fertility specialist. With psychotherapy, Virgilia was able to work through some very painful, yet empowering, discussions with her practitioner about her own childhood, her time in the womb and her parent's background. Virgilia, in addition, found comfort in the support of the flower essences that gave her the strength, the courage and the insights to make the best use of her psychotherapy sessions. Five years later, Virgilia had, still, not conceived but her heart remained open to the possibility of doing so. Virgilia, however, was, now, no longer so desperate, she felt much healthier in body and mind and, most importantly, she had understood the reasons why this time in her life had been so difficult for her.

Virgilia became profoundly inspired by her past experiences and, now, works as a flower essence consultant with women, and their partners, who are trying to conceive. Virgilia has, also, developed her own range of essences and essential oils for fertility enhancement and miscarriage. Virgilia's measure of success can be seen when her client and her partner are able to take back some degree of control into their lives and to feel able to live more joyously and with some sense of fulfillment, irrespective of whether they become parents. Virgilia is, now, creating the products and doing the work that she so wished that she could have done in the past. Virgilia cannot predict whether she and her partner will ever become parents but, somehow, using her experience to help others in one of the most emotionally-charged of life's experiences, and one that is so little openly discussed, has brought meaning to her own tragic feelings of pain and loss.

Let's take an example – Jacquenetta's story

Jacquenetta was inspired by acupuncture as a result of undertaking some life-changing personal therapy herself. Jacquenetta's personal therapy had the big-bang effect on her and she yearned to learn all about it and to practice acupuncture and Chinese medicine herself.

While Jacquenetta was undertaking her preliminary training course, and as she first began to practice, she realized, at a profound personal level, what an amazing tool acupuncture could be for healing many ills. Jacquenetta was, also, fascinated by the whole topic of the mind-body concept and the simple way in which it works. From this launching pad, Jacquenetta believed that she could work at something that she enjoyed enormously and that she could simultaneously make a difference to the lives of others.

Fired up with enthusiasm, Jacquenetta set out on her intended mission and was able to seek advice, when necessary, in order to surmount the many obstacles that inevitably were strewn in her path. Jacquenetta, like many practitioners, overcame the hump of dwindling financial resources while her business was being established. Jacquenetta, also, found herself struggling with the self-blame syndrome whereby she chastised herself for any perceived failures and feared being over-obliging with her client. Jacquenetta, of course, rode the wave of having to deal with the massive psychological issues that arose within her as a result of the nature of her work. Eventually, the passage of time and the accumulation of experience, together with a dogged determination to succeed, allowed Jacquenetta to overcome her many obstacles. Now Jacquenetta has an established practice and she receives constant satisfaction from her work because she had what it took to weather the storm.

How would you be evolving yourself?

Will you notice the way in which you might naturally be evolving with your client? Your new-found vocation may seem perfect and you may be inspirationally motivated to accomplish great things. This utopian state may, regretfully, not last forever but, maybe, now, you can regard the ups and downs as part of your evolutionary passage.

How will you be looking after yourself?

It may often be vital to remind yourself that, in order to help others, you must, first and foremost, care for yourself and you must take a dose of your own medicine. The pitfalls for you may be that you could go over the top in terms of your mission in life and, as a result, you could seriously neglect yourself in the process. Sometimes when you decide to assist others, you might, amazingly, forget to help yourself. This may be an obvious and over-worked cliché but it holds as much water today as it is did when the phrase was first coined. If you focus exclusively on helping yourself and on gaining your job-satisfaction, then, your client will automatically benefit. Try being selfish for a change and appreciate how beneficial it can be for all those in your orbit and beyond.

The most significant point to appreciate here may be that it will be imperative for you to help yourself before you can ever, possibly, even dream of assisting another. Regardless of your particular therapeutic discipline, the ideal for you would be to sample a whole range of alternative practices in order to heal your mind, body, biochemistry and spirituality because any disharmony will have arisen from your life's experience, distress, ill-health and personal hardship. What you may constantly fail to appreciate, however, might be that your personal in-depth investigation, and its resolution, will be a life-affirming and evolutionary necessity for you as a practitioner. Personal evolution will certainly be essential for you if you are to lead a happy, healthy and successful life and to fulfill your ultimate potential both personally and professionally. It may not always be possible, of course, for you to find the time, the energy and the finances to undertake and to continue formal therapeutic advancement with another practitioner. The best policy may, then, be for you to strike a middle course and not to feel despondent if you, temporarily, stray off your healing path. Sometimes you may be able to negotiate a discounted rate for your own personal therapy from a colleague or even to arrange to swap treatments with a trusted peer.

Be aware that when hell-bent on a mission of self-enlightenment and health-recovery, you could, of course, find yourself becoming over-keen. You may, for instance, become ludicrously over-zealous or overflowing with dogged determination. Content yourself with the news that it may simply be where you are right now, but the way you are, currently, will soon change. Often, when you give yourself permission to be yourself, you will naturally evolve as a dynamic practitioner. Learn to listen to your inner adviser who will tell you all that you will need to know about yourself.

There will inevitably be times when being a helper can amount to far too much and what may be worse is that the warning signs will often creep up unnoticed and quite insidiously. Perhaps one of the greatest challenges of being a therapeutic practitioner may be knowing when to stop and to take a break.

Ask yourself ...

Are you allowing yourself to develop and to evolve naturally in accordance with the dictates of your inner self? Have you sampled a cross-spectrum of therapeutic practices in order to deal with your most fundamental issues? Do you automatically know when to book some additional personal therapy or some self-care? Do you firmly believe that investigation into yourself will be of enormous benefit to you personally? Can you concede that looking at your own psychological issues would assist you with your clients? Would you like to say good-bye to your aches and pains, your frequent malaise and your comfort-seeking habits? Would it not be time, now, to rid yourself of your chronic indigestion, your high blood-pressure, your heart palpitations or your sporadic asthma? Do you really consider that personal therapy would be a waste of your time or are you simply wishing earnestly to evade your own painful issues? Why would you wish to deny yourself an opportunity to relieve yourself of emotional baggage, physical discomfort and the general pain of life? Do you still sit with one foot in the allopathic camp? Are you really dealing with those issues that arise from your interaction with your client? Would the services of a supervisor or a mentor resolve a whole collection of problems that may be arising within you? Have you spoken to a range of practitioners in other fields about their work? Do you feel yourself to be on a mission because you can think of nothing else but your work?

Let's take an example – Oberon's story

Oberon works as a shamanic healer who has made contact with a number of practitioners in his area in order to provide support, to exchange ideas and to promote his own business through client-referrals. Oberon finds that most of his work-related problems can, thus, be solved by contact with fellow-practitioners and by problem-solving with like-minded people.

As a shamanic healer, Oberon uses power-animals in order to access his own healing powers. Early on in his training, Oberon discovered his most trusted companion and his fellow-healer in the form of his power-animal, the cougar, with whom he has, now, worked for a number of years. Oberon uses this powerful guide when he is beset by indecision or when he does not know how to proceed with his client. On one occasion, Oberon noticed that his cougar jumped when he was about to make a mistake when applying healing to one of his clients. From this moment on, Oberon appreciated the strength and the wisdom of such a healing guide. Oberon, thus, learned not only to trust his cougar implicitly but also to rely solely on his own instincts and his personal intuition. Once this working relationship had been established with his cougar, Oberon, then, found that many of his clients were simultaneously able to make a direct contact with their own personal power-animals and to benefit from the relationship that became firmly recognized.

Would you wish to be a saver of souls?

Will you be hell-bent on a heaven-sent healing mission with your client? As a practitioner, you may, perhaps, feel as if you are on a healing crusade, particularly if you have benefited enormously from being the recipient of such life-transforming therapy yourself. Being a practitioner, however, does not mean that you should be a saver of souls at the expense of your own wellbeing and your inherent peace of mind.

What will be your healing mission?

If your own healing journey has led you along a joyous path, you may feel inclined to prostate yourself in the furtherance of your healing destiny. Your earnest desire to help others can be highly admirable but, occasionally, you could be at risk from getting carried away with being too beneficent. By all means be a dedicated and a responsible professional but do not make yourself a doormat for your client because neither of you will benefit from this approach. Often the doormat-syndrome will blossom because of your humble self-esteem that will usually accompany the kind of adversity that had initially brought you into the therapeutic arena.

Remember always to put yourself at the top of your own agenda and, consequently, every client you see will benefit enormously from your wise attitude. Your first duty should be to yourself and, when you care lovingly for yourself, you will, then, be able to help others effortlessly. As the catalyst for your client's healing journey, you will need to be in good shape yourself in order to do such a job. Rest here to consider whether you are helping others at the expense of assisting yourself.

Ask yourself . . .

Could you believe that you have been given a special mission from on high? Will you feel that you must persuade others to benefit from your enlightenment? Do you consider that you alone can help that lame dog over the style? Do you earnestly want to bring more souls into the light and would you go to the ends of the earth in order to do so? Would you travel across the globe in order to save a few wanderers from the fire and brimstone? Are you keen to heal the entire planet and the rest of the universe in one lifetime? Do you feel that because of your privileges you must, now, be a crusader? Would you wish to be a shining example to your client and your colleague? Will you consider that you should make some humble sacrifices, now, because of your own miraculous recovery experiences? Will your life utterly fall apart if your client does not become an exponent of the cause? Are you over-caring for others as a means of under-caring for yourself and, thus, deflecting the limelight away from your own problems?

Let's look at it another way – Buying a new car

A man goes out one day to purchase a brand-new car. The prospective buyer knows that the car is a good buy because he has sought advice from several reliable, knowledgeable and independent parties before proceeding with the purchase. The man has, also, read several impartial reports of the car's excellent performance and reliability. The buyer goes to the car-showroom with optimism and with excitement. The car has been thoroughly tested and has been given the quality-control seal of approval before it can leave the showroom with its proud, new owner. *The car is bright and shiny new without a mark, a scratch or a speck of dust on it and it comes with a full tank of petrol. The new owner feels as if he has died and gone to heaven.*

The car's new owner will, now, be at a fork in the road in terms of his relationship with his vehicle. The new purchaser may drive cautiously, may valet his car lovingly, may service it regularly, may park it carefully and will ensure that it has been topped up with petrol before any long journey. All who travel in the vehicle will find the experience comfortable, safe and pleasurable. The car will reflect the owner's pride in himself and his possessions as well as being evidence of his sound wisdom with regard to his investment in this means of transport.

An alternative scenario may ensue with a neglectful owner. The man may take the car from the showroom, may hurtle down the freeway and, perhaps, will risk a crash. The owner may allow his car to get dirty in no time at all. The car-owner may, also, neglect to service his new car at the recommended times. The car may get scratched easily because its owner will park it at a funny angle or it may be stolen because he will forget to lock it up sensibly. Often the owner will not remember to put petrol into his car and so frequently he will get stranded in out-of-the way places. This will upset the driver's passengers and will cause him much inconvenience and embarrassment. When it comes to selling this car, of course, it will not be given a clean bill of health for the next prospective purchaser. What would you do if you owned this car and in which car would you prefer to travel?

Would you wish to be an evangelist?

Will you feel that you have been given a directive from on high in order to preach the gospel to your client? You may feel that you should, henceforth, beat the drum on behalf of the world and be a gospel-preacher for your profession. You will, almost certainly, harbor such feelings, in some guise, but beware of letting your convictions get out of control.

How will you spread the immortal word?

Because of your own personal road-to-Damascus experience with alternative therapy, you may feel that you have been charged with the responsibility of spreading the sacred word. By all means advertise your services with conviction and with enthusiasm but do not become a preacher to the masses. You can only be of use to your client if she wishes to be assisted by you.

When you come face to face with the troubled man in the street, your halo may begin to glow. You may feel prompted to give this distressed soul the benefit of your experience. Do not, however, let your halo become tarnished by your own desire to enlighten the world. You cannot impose therapy on the unwary or the unwilling. Usually the man in the street will not be that interested in the amazing discoveries that you have made and he may, possibly, resent you for assiduously imposing your view on him. You may feel tempted to become a walking publicity agent for your therapeutic discipline but you cannot change the thinking and the cultural programming of the uninitiated overnight. Pause for a moment to consider the traps that may be strewn in your path if you become over-evangelical about your therapeutic treatment. You may believe that your mission should be to advertise the services of your profession to everyone with whom you come into contact. Do not, however, become so intoxicated with your own beliefs and your personal enthusiasm to the extent that you may rob others of any free choice in the matter.

Ask yourself . . .

Do you feel that you should convert the man in the paper-shop down the road because he really could do with some flower essences or a touch of spiritual healing? Might you consider that the girl next door could do with some counseling in order to deal with her fear of spiders? Would you desperately like to get your hands on that guy in the office who has a crippling arthritic condition and, subsequently, show him the way? Do you think that by giving an advertising leaflet to every pregnant woman in the street you will convert all would-be mothers for all time to natural childbirth? Will you want to forbid Auntie May from taking antibiotics and desire to give her a stern lecture on suppressive drugs? Perhaps your friend cannot be converted to the cause and should be left to make her own way in life? Possibly your neighbor's views are so entrenched in orthodox doctrine that it would take more than a quick chitchat from you to change those opinions? Do you really think that Mr Average could understand alternative philosophy by a chance remark that you might make? Do you sincerely believe that you could encourage that man to alter his entire belief system, reprogram his thinking and adopt an entirely new lifestyle because you have, now, told him the truth? Would that woman really be prepared to give up everything for which she has lived for many decades just because you tell her that there might be an alternative way of life? Will there be any point in boring a whole load of people at a party with your diatribe on erroneous medical thinking, together with your opus magnum on the wonders of alternative healing practice?

Let's look at it another way – The double-glazing salesman

You have had a long and arduous day at the chalk-face at work. You stagger home and hurriedly rustle up something to eat. You put your feet up and you manage to get a bit of much-needed shut-eye. Peace and quiet reigns at last. The phone rings, however, and your dreams are instantly shattered. Some well-intended salesman, now, attempts to sell you Sparkling Wonder double-glazing.

Well actually your house does tend to be a little cold in the winter and the traffic outside can be noisy. Being an intelligent being, however, you are able to make up your own mind about home-improvements. Your bank balance, of course, may not be that healthy and a further overdraft would not be greeted with delight by your bank manager. You could do with a holiday, if you had the ready cash, and this might be infinitely preferably to smartening up your windows. Nevertheless, right now, all you want to do is to curl up, to eat supper and to have a snooze. Because you wish to adhere to social etiquette, however, you politely say "Not just now, thank you". But still the salesman persists in trying to demolish your protests. The salesman continues by arguing the economic sense of the project, by attempting to understand your situation and by perpetually probing about your personal circumstances. You start to fume inwardly and begin to feel compromised. This man may be trading on your good nature and he will be trying to pull at all your guilt-strings. Would, now, be the right time to slam the phone down?

Actually this double-glazing salesman will really only be interested in getting a sale and in earning his commission. The salesman will, in fact, not be at all concerned with your need for a holiday, your impending financial ruin or the fact that your meager supper may rapidly be getting cold. The salesman may, by chance, believe wholeheartedly in the efficacy of his prod-

*uct but he has not, in any way, considered life from your perspective. Would
you really wish to become a double-glazing salesman?*

Would you wish to be a one-way street merchant?

Will you ever concede that there could be several alternative
routes to general health improvement for your client? With any
life-changing self-discovery that you may have just undergone,
you may, now, feel that your chosen journey should obviously be
the right one for everyone.

How many paths will lead to the end of the road?

It would be perfectly natural for you to consider that you
have found the ultimate key to your therapeutic success and that
the rest of the world should benefit from your most significant
discovery. Remember, however, that your path may have been
absolutely right for you but it may not be the correct alternative
route for your client.

If you have taken the physical route to health improvement,
and not focused too much on shifting your emotional baggage,
do not consider that this route should be adopted by your client.
If you have found a remedy-oriented route to optimal health, do
not attempt to convince your client that she can only find success
by this means herself. Your client should be allowed to follow her
own route towards therapeutic resolution. It will be important
for you to respect your client's wishes and, if possible, to envisage her viewpoint. Your client, moreover, may not actually have
the tenacity or the courage to travel to the ends of the earth in
order to resolve her emotional, physical, spiritual and biochemical toxicity as you might have done.

Indeed, your client may well come around to your way of
thinking eventually, after making one or two mistakes along the
way, but she should be permitted to draw her own conclusions,
unaided, without any arm-wrestling tactics from you. Your client
should be given the opportunity to learn from her own experiences. Your client should, furthermore, be free to make her own
decisions as a person in her own right without being reminded
with the "I-told-you-so" routine. Holding a baby's hand will not
ensure that he will learn to walk speedily and successfully. Do not

take this responsibility on yourself and do not blame yourself if your client elects to walk her own path, whatever the outcome. Trust that your client will be the only one who knows what could work for her and allow her to receive this gift.

Ask yourself . . .

Does your client, maybe, want to take matters more slowly and to tackle her problem from a spiritual rather than from a physical angle? Does your client, possibly, feel that the nutritional approach should be at the top of her agenda rather than your touch-oriented therapy? Would your client really be an extrovert and, so, will not warm easily to reflective thinking or to heavy psychotherapeutic probing? Will your client not actually be interested in her trauma from past lives but will merely wish to acquire some stress-reduction techniques for everyday use right now? Will your client be quite obviously nervous about a computer-based diagnosis using bioresonance technology? Does your client feel that she only needs a holding-mechanism, now, that will suffice for the present at least? Would your client, perhaps, not be inclined to attend your practice regularly for the next year or so? Will your client, in essence, be capable of any in-depth soul-searching and, consequently, of facing her true emotions? Will your client be really ready and fully able to face the stark truth about her condition and will she be well equipped to tackle the consequences of dealing with it? Would it be inappropriate for your client to fast for three months, or to drink her own urine every morning for the rest of her life, in order to promote good health?

Let's look at it another way – There are many roads to Rome

If you wish to make a journey to Rome, the city of culture, you will be beset with many choices and decisions. You could, for instance, travel with all speed by air provided, of course, that you are not phobic about flying. You would obviously need to be able to get to an airport that offers reasonably-convenient flights to Rome. Maybe there will not be a convenient airport near you and this will make your decision easier. If you can get to an airport, then, you will need to decide how you could travel there. Could you drive yourself and park safely at the airport for the duration of your journey? Will your car be scraped, knocked, raided, vandalized or stolen while you are away? Could you get a friend to drive you to the airport? Maybe you do not have any friends? Would a taxi-ride be prohibitively expensive or out of all proportion to the cut-price airfare that you have just secured?

Would it be better to drive all the way to Rome? You could drive to the coast and, then, get a ferry across to Europe? Provided that you do not live in the Antarctic or Tasmania, this might be a viable option. Will your sea-crossing be stormy when you decide to travel? The ferry-crossing may be cheaper than a flight or, maybe, not. You would need to buy some maps, of course, in order to negotiate the road through France, Switzerland, Austria and/or Slovenia and, then, Italy itself. Will you take the quick but expensive auto-route or will you decide to stick to the slow yet scenic country roads? Will your drive be pleasant and hassle-free or will you drive flat out all the way to your destination and, then, arrive a little jaded? Perhaps, after all, you should consider going by coach?

Maybe you could travel by train across Europe? Would the train fare be above your budget or do you not give a damn about the expense? The train journey may mean that you will need to change trains many times and to co-ordinate your interconnections carefully. Will the train take the strain out of your journey or will it be tedious and will it demand uncomfortable overnight accommodation?

Well, perhaps, it would be better to go by boat all the way? You could go on a cruise right around to the Mediterranean and dock at the foot of Italy or at the toe of Sicily? Cruise-ships are great and it would be like a holiday, in itself, before you even get to Rome. But, maybe, you would become seasick or, possibly, claustrophobic in your cabin? Would you need to hire a car, to take the train or to hire a coach to reach your final destination? Maybe you should contemplate hitch-hiking?

Will you remember to take your passport, your travelers' cheques, your currency, your credit cards and your insurance documentation? After all this contemplation and planning, would it not be better to consider staying at home? Will your personal decisions be based on time-constraints, finances, travel options, phobic limitations and personal preferences? You can be sure that your choices will not be precisely the same as some of your fellow-travelers. Will your decisions be right for you, even if you do have to learn by experience and, then, take an alternative route next time? How will you get to your ultimate destination?

PART 3
YOU AND YOUR BUSINESS

10 HOW WOULD YOU LAUNCH YOUR PRACTICE?

Where would you be going in life?

Will you have looked at the weather forecast lately before floating your practice? It will always be important for you to consider where your career path might be taking you as this will form a part of your unique self-development plan. As a practitioner, you should be aware that you might never have embarked on your career unless it would be of significant therapeutic benefit to you personally and you should not be ashamed to acknowledge this vital point.

When will you wish to start your practice?

Deciding when the time will be right for you to launch your ship will be a strategic move on your part. If you are a fledgling practitioner or a trainee, you, maybe, cannot wait to plunge into your future career with blazing enthusiasm and with unparalleled zeal. You may have a burning passion to get started in your new role. You might regard it as a shameful waste of all your time, your heartache and your money if you are not instantly putting what you have learned into practice. Perhaps you will be counting the days until you are fully qualified, although be patient because your time will eventually come.

Alternatively, you may be reluctant and will want to put off the evil day when you will finally need to launch your practice.

Be kind to yourself, however, and start only when you are truly ready. You may wish to consider your position if you find yourself dragging your feet, in any way, with regard to your starting work. If you do intend to practice, at some point, you will, of course, need to jump in and get on with the job. The only way of learning the business, and the tricks of the trade, will be by actually getting your feet wet.

Ask yourself . . .

Do you feel reticent about taking the plunge and becoming a working professional? Do you feel reluctant to talk to others of your intention to set up in business as a practitioner? Would you have every intention of entering therapeutic practice but simply cannot muster the energy to get your business launched right now? Maybe you have, now, at last, discovered your true mission in life and will want to start banging the drum with gusto? Do you consider that you have finally discovered what you really want to do in life as a profession? Do you feel impatient to get going with your work and long to see some clients?

When will you finally start your practice?

The secret of becoming a successful practitioner will be to get your timing right in terms of launching your business. If you are a newly-qualified practitioner and fully intend to set up in practice, for instance, you might feel totally unfit to undertake your work immediately after completing your training course. When you qualify, the temptation may, then, be to run out immediately and to take another training course in the vain hope that the second time around will deliver the goods. You might, also, buy a lorry load of books and burn some midnight oil. These panic tactics are not uncommon on graduation but why not simply let your occupation develop as a natural component of your evolutionary process?

Some would-be practitioners may teeter on the brink or never actually get going. If you come into this category, then, worry not. The secret will be to remember that taking a practitioner's training course will be a part of your personal, evolutionary development and, perhaps, this action will be all that you may require for that purpose. You may not wish to start your practice immediately after graduation, therefore, or you may not wish to become a practitioner at all. If that might be what you want, or what seems to be happening, then, go with the flow and give yourself permission to be yourself.

If you definitely do not wish to join the therapist's brigade, then, merely go out and conquer the world as you would wish to seize it and give not another thought to being a healer. If you have, at last, found your true self by taking a therapeutic training course, then, merely thank the universe for having found a creative way of showing you how to fulfill your destiny. Now will certainly not be the time for bosom-beating but rather an occasion for celebration and the acceptance of fond memories of an enlightening wakeup call. Your time, your money and your effort will have obviously been well spent because you have discovered your truly-divine path. It will not be obligatory for you to take a professional training course and, then, automatically to become a full-time practitioner for the rest of your days.

Ask yourself . . .

Are you ready to start your business practice right now? Can you be content with starting your professional work when you feel completely ready to do so? Do you feel ill-equipped for the job and do you lack the confidence in your ability to work as a practitioner? Do you feel as if you ought to take another training course, or the same classes all over again, in order to feel confident enough to start up your practice? Are you wavering because crunch-time has ultimately arrived? Have you decided that you will find another way of fulfilling your potential? Do you feel as if you have obtained all you need out of your training course and, so, you do not feel inclined to set up in practice at all? Have you suddenly realized that you would actually prefer to become an airline pilot, a tightrope artiste or a politician? Do you, now, feel free enough to hire a boat and to sail around the world? Can you give yourself permission to fulfill your own destiny, in your own way, without any pangs of conscience?

Let's take an example – Titania's story

Titania had a full-time job as a nurse before she decided to retrain as a homeopathic practitioner. Once qualified, Titania wanted to work full-time as a practitioner but seemed wedded to the salary that accompanied her daytime job. Eventually, Titania started in practice on a part-time basis by just seeing a few clients in the evenings and at weekends. This halfway house, unfortunately, then, meant that Titania was torn between doing what earned her a crust and doing what she really wanted to do in life. Titania, thus, began to suffer the anguish and the disappointment of not fulfilling her destiny while, at the same time, wearing herself out and worrying about earning money.

An important shift in Titania's thinking occurred as the number of her clients grew and her yearning to let go of her former nursing career took a firm hold. It seemed that this mental adjustment was the key to what Titania really needed in order to launch her business. Moreover, promoting her business became a natural instinct for Titania and this inclination paid handsome dividends. At this point, the number of clients that were attracted to Titania seemed to magically grow even more because she was, now, focused full-time on living and being a practitioner. Consequently, Titania's need for financial security was met by her dedication to doing what gave her the greatest job-satisfaction.

Will you wish to continue your practice?

If you are an established practitioner, you will, quite regularly, need to review your vocation. Any self-questioning or doubtful thoughts about continuing in practice that you may be secretly harboring will all be perfectly natural, healthy and only to be expected. This phenomenon may be regarded as keeping an open mind and ensuring that the work you are doing will be exactly in line with your aspirations. Being a doormat because you think you ought to be a martyr will not be, at all, beneficial for you or for your client.

If, one of these bright days, you decide that you no longer wish to continue in practice, then, just go with the flow. Becoming a fully-fledged practitioner does not mean that you have signed the pledge for eternity. You might, moreover, be advised to regularly review whether you actually wish to remain in practice, or even to radically alter the way in which you work, every so often. If you feel inclined to work in another field, to take an early retirement, or simply to take an extended break, then, do so. Again this type of decision will be an important part of your evolutionary journey and should be acknowledged and greeted as such by you.

Ask yourself . . .

    Do you still look forward to seeing your next client with as much relish and enthusiasm as you did on the day when you first started work? Does your work give you endless joy and job-satisfaction or has the daily grind become a tedious drudge? Have you realized that one-to-one therapy has too narrow a focus for your particular talents? Perhaps your heart will not be in your work any longer and fresher fields might beckon? Maybe your attitude to your work has, now, gone quite stale? Do you feel that you, possibly, need more time for yourself? Have you given too much of yourself already and, now, you do not wish to continue as a therapeutic practitioner? Do you want to devote your life exclusively to helping others? Possibly you have enough money with which to retire from gainful employment? Maybe that trip around the globe appears to be more pressing than seeing a regular caseload of clients every week? Are you skating dangerously near to burnout and do you feel that you should, now, bow gracefully out of the game? Perhaps it would be wise to question your vocation and your need to do therapeutic work, at least, once in a while?

Let's take an example – Hippolyta's story

    Hippolyta took a number of practitioner's training courses in rapid succession within the space of 5 or 6 years. Hippolyta, first, studied massage and reiki healing as a means of introducing herself to the concept of self-healing. Spurred on by her quest for self-enlightenment, Hippolyta, next, turned to craniosacral therapy and this allowed her to take an in-depth look at herself and stirred up much mud from the depths of her soul. Hippolyta's training in craniosacral therapy was, also, underpinned by several years of being the recipient of this therapeutic treatment. Because Hippolyta, still, felt that there was unfinished business in her soul, she, then, took a course in counseling almost immediately after finishing her craniosacral course. Again, Hippolyta's counseling training was supported by a countless number of therapeutic sessions as part of her preparation for practice.

    Needless to say, Hippolyta was exhausted by the time that she had finished her various training courses and had undergone her own personal therapy as part of her induction to live practice. Hippolyta had, in consequence, reached a turning point in her life. After seeing a handful of clients, Hippolyta realized that she had achieved for herself everything that she wanted in the therapeutic vein. Hippolyta concluded that she had needed to look into herself thoroughly and had gone all out for her personal goal but, at the same time, she realized that to live the life of a practitioner no longer held the magic for her.

Hippolyta, thus, decided to delay starting her practice while keeping an open mind about her future occupation. A number of different options for business activities have floated through Hippolyta's mind but living with indecision and uncertainty has, now, become possible for her.

How would you light the touch-paper?

Will you be prepared to invest time, money and enthusiasm into launching your business? You should, of course, carefully consider the run-up to starting in practice as a therapeutic practitioner. You might, very profitably, spend some time mulling over the preliminary arrangements that you will be required to make before ultimately floating your business.

Will you wish to forge ahead?

Long before that auspicious occasion arrived when you were presented with your qualifying diploma, perhaps, your mind will have begun to work overtime in anticipation of the road ahead. This enthusiasm can be regarded as a sign of your commitment to the therapeutic work that you have decided to undertake. In devoting time to an exercise of forethought, you will, also, find yourself experiencing the excitement and the anticipation that can drive you relentlessly forward. With the right degree of fervor, you will, consequently, be fired up to get your business off the ground as if your life depended upon it.

Always ensure, nonetheless, that your zeal does not get entirely out of hand and become desperation. Fraught-thinking can lead you to desperate measures and will muddle your mind. Fretfulness, moreover, can insidiously convey itself to your potential client who may not want to consult someone who appears to be panic-stricken or effusively over-enthusiastic.

Ask yourself . . .
Are you really fired up with enthusiasm and almost impatient to crank up the engine? Do you find that your inspiration simply flows and

the ideas just arrive when you require them? Have you devoted enough time to examining the way in which you should launch your practice? Can you put your individual stamp on the process of setting yourself up in business? How do you view the prospect of self-employment as a practitioner in private practice? Have you managed to secure a paid position for your work as a therapeutic practitioner and, therefore, you do not need to work privately? Will you need to retain your day-job temporarily or indefinitely? Can you stop and take stock before you plunge headlong into the abyss?

Will you wish to hold yourself back?

You may realize that your enthusiasm will inevitably be coupled with many reservations that may accompany your business launch. Such trepidation will be perfectly natural and almost to be expected of you. Launching a new business, in an unknown area, can be charged with emotion and, thus, may often not be an easy task for you. Allow yourself, therefore, to examine your motivations in order to avoid the pitfalls that could be associated with launching and running a private therapeutic practice.

If you are in any doubt about the way in which you could tackle the job, ask several other established practitioners about the way in which their practice was launched. By this means, you can take the weight off your mind and some of the worry out of the equation for yourself. Pick the brains of other successful professionals who can stimulate your ideas, by all means, but ensure that you tackle the setup task in your way. Remember that launching your ship will be a personal statement but that you can, in addition, feed off the experience of those who have trodden this well-worn trail before.

Ask yourself . . .

Do you feel a healthy mixture of trepidation and excitement at the prospect of launching your business? Do you constantly feel that you are not ready for the off in terms of launching your rocket? Could there be something that you are not quite getting around to doing? Do you feel that there could be just something else that you may need to do before you get down to planning your promotional campaign? Are you putting off finding accommodation, designing promotional material or completing your training course? Do you believe that self-employment can be an ex-

citing realm or a daunting prospect? Are you rushing ahead too speedily and should you really be taking things step by step? Do you believe that plunging in at the deep end must be the best move?

Let's take an example – Juliet's story

Juliet had difficulty initially in finding somewhere suitable in which to practice as a medical herbalist. Juliet was keen to start her work and did not want any logistic problems to hold her up. First, Juliet hired a room in a beauty therapy clinic but soon found that the location was not really appropriate for her. Juliet simply did not feel comfortable about the work ambiance and, therefore, decided to seek a new practice location.

Juliet, next, found what she initially thought was an ideal location in a remote farmhouse that was both quiet and peaceful. The atmosphere of this locality was pleasant and the owner of the premises was friendly, encouraging and helpful. The fly in this ointment, however, was that the entrance to the building was difficult to find. At one point, some distinctive landmarks were placed by the entrance and these served as a guide to newcomers. However, these directional aids were later removed and Juliet could not persuade anyone to reinstate them. The result of this catastrophe was that some of Juliet's clients could not find her easily and, so, promptly gave up or did not wish to travel to such a remote area. Juliet, therefore, was personally happy with her secluded location but her prospective clients were obviously not.

Finally, Juliet decided that she would work from home and she arranged her living accommodation accordingly. Juliet was, at first, concerned about working from home but, then, used some visualization techniques in order to convince herself that she could make it work. Working from home, thus, was the answer to this particular problem for Juliet and, moreover, it suited her purse as well as accommodating her comfort-factor.

What would you need to get started?

Will you be able to predict the pace of your future when establishing your practice? Once you are under starter's orders, you may simply propel yourself forward as soon as the gun has been fired. Sometimes, of course, you may need a gentle push even after the engines have been fired up. This seeming intransigence should not be interpreted by you as a sign of a calamity but merely seen as a natural phenomenon related to the laws of motion.

How will you envisage the road ahead?

Getting your life into perspective can often provide the magic formula that will set you on your way. If you pause for a moment in order to consider how far you have traveled, you will realize that the road ahead may not, then, seem so daunting.

Every moment of your life has brought you to where you are now. If you can look over your shoulder, you will see that the highway on which you have just traveled has not always been straight and direct. You may have scaled mountains or waded through swirling rivers. You may have crossed the desert or hacked your way through the jungle. You may have traveled in good weather when the going was easy or you may have had to plough through storm, hail, snow and wind. The conditions may be a bit similar, too, on the journey ahead.

Your journey forward may take you through the meadows or by the stream. Your voyage may take you through tunnels or across bridges. Your excursion may lead you uphill and down dale. The going may be tough, on some occasions, but could be more undulating, at other times. The weather may sometimes be fine and sunny and the path ahead of you may be clear. You may, however, encounter a hurricane or become windswept and, occasionally, you will need to weather a freak storm. You may get soaked to the skin in the process but you will soon dry out. The road ahead may be clear, when visibility is good on a cloudless day, and you will know exactly which route to take. Sometimes, of course, you will not be able to see further than the end of your nose when visibility is poor. At this juncture simply pause for rest and, of course, you will need to have time-out periodically.

The route may often be perfectly straight and your journey will simply happen without any intervention from you. You may frequently never be able to see around the next bend and, therefore, you will not know what to expect. This is life and, so, accept it in all its glory. Some mishaps you may be able to avoid or to circumvent. Other hazards may be beyond your scope to control or to manipulate in your favor. Accept that life consists of unpredictability and living with that knowledge can be a good lesson in personal survival.

Ask yourself . . .

Are you all ready to go but will you need to give a thought to how you are going to begin? Will you be prepared for the ups and downs of launching your business? Can you reflect on what has gone by in the past? Can you imagine a secure and enjoyable future? Do you believe that all will be straightforward and that your clients will simply flock to your door? Do you secretly fear that you may not make the grade as a working professional? Can you get started in business and worry about the consequences later? Can you, now, live with uncertainty for the fore-seeable future?

Let's take an example – Phoebe's story

Phoebe trained as a psychotherapist but her greatest concern about being in practice was that she would become lost for words with her client and that she would not have a solution to any problem in a tricky situation. Phoebe's fear was so great that it prevented her from setting up in practice for well over a year after she had qualified.

Phoebe's first paying client, unfortunately, happened to open up the floodgates for her by directly reflecting her own fears. Phoebe's client had consulted her for problems concerned with public speaking and with giving a presentation in front of an audience. This was a predicament that Phoebe herself had battled with for some years. Phoebe's client, however, marked a turning point for her in her career and in her attitude to working. When the sessions with her client began, Phoebe started to realize what role fear had to play in ruling her own psychological roost but reassured herself with the inner knowledge that she could be of some help to her client. Self-belief was a hard lesson that Phoebe was required to learn. Phoebe soon appreciated that all the fears that she had harbored about being a self-supporting practitioner were direct reflections of her own childhood wounds and traumas. Phoebe's reservations, in fact, were all centered on her feelings and her negative beliefs about not being capable, not knowing enough and not being good enough.

One day everything clicked into place for Phoebe and she started to feel adequate, competent and skilled. The crunch came when Phoebe's life took a dramatic change of direction and she learned how accurate her intuition could be and the way in which she could put it to work.

Phoebe's reliance on her intuitive powers became strongly apparent and this, subsequently, gave her an unbridled confidence. At this juncture, Phoebe's clients began to come out of the woodwork and practical considerations that had previously hampered her, like finding a practice location or purchasing a reclining chair, simply slotted into place.

How much might you think you would be worth?

Will you under-sell yourself on the open market when launching your business? One of the surest ways of putting yourself down, and ensuring that you stay there, will be not to charge enough money for the services that you offer. There may be much justification on your part for not charging the going rate but it may all amount to an I-am-not-good-enough syndrome.

Where will you be in your self-estimation equation?

The world, as it exists today, can be a topsy-turvy place to say the very least. The stockbroker, the pop-idol or the Harley Street surgeon will earn a fortune, will drive a flashy car and may own a yacht moored in a fashionable marina in the Mediterranean. In a non-upside-down world, the professionals who would be worshipped and highly respected would be the therapeutic fraternity. The rest of the population would be earning peanuts and fishing for compliments.

As a qualified practitioner, you will bring to your client a lifetime's worth of experience with, perhaps, years of struggle, decades of misery and your personal ability to overcome ill-health, hardship and suffering. You will offer to your client a unique opportunity to follow your example, to partake of the gift of freedom from pain and to emerge into a healthier and more contented way of life. This will be the greatest gift you could ever, possibly, give to anyone on the planet and, so, it would be utterly unthinkable for you to charge less than an adequate fee for your invaluable services. It may be criminal even to think that market forces have a say in the matter at all. It may be a tragic indictment of the so-called modern world that society has not yet realized and not yet applauded the true value of members of the alternative therapeutic community. All alternative practitioners should, in reality, be charging ten times the sum currently regarded as the norm by society. But, sadly, we live in an unenlightened and an unfair world.

Being a member of the alternative caring profession in to-day's society may, of course, mean that you might feel that you should give your services for less than the standard rate, or even for nothing, on occasion. This will be the most ludicrous way of thinking and, should you be tempted to even contemplate such folly, then, you will surely need to take a long hard look at your motivations and your self-image. Charging a meager fee, or none at all, for your services will debase your self-esteem. In addition, this tack will do nothing for your client who should be taking full responsibility for facing up to the kinds of issues that will con-tribute to her ill-health. It will, therefore, be a sheer disservice to your client, as well as being a crime to deprive yourself of what you truly deserve, by being poorly paid for the most valuable contribution that anyone could ever make to society today.

Ask yourself . . .

Do you charge a meager fee because you consider that no-one would ever want to pay the full whack for you? Do you consider that you are less competent than your colleague in the next room who may be more experienced and, therefore, you feel you should charge less? Do you find yourself extending the time allotted to your client because you feel guilty about charging her so much money? Are you tempted to give your client some extra time because you feel ashamed about charging her anything at all? Do you catch yourself giving free therapy over the phone as a means of compensating for the fee you would normally charge your client? Do you feel that your client might be a bit hard up and, so, you tend to feel sorry for her? Do you think that your fee reflects the hard work that you have put into gaining your qualifications? Do you believe that you are not really working hard because you enjoy your work? Do you charge a low rate because you secretly consider that you are not really very good at your job? Do you have a number of self-punishing syndromes still alive and kicking in your psyche? Are you reluctant to ask your client for money at the end of her session? Does your client ever manage to escape without paying your fee? Can you compare your fee with the price of alcohol, cigarettes, packaged holidays, running a car, social drugs and supermarket food?

Let's take an example – Bianca's story

For Bianca, a health kinesiologist, the main obstacle to launching her practice was having the courage to spend money on advertising and to charge a respectable fee. Bianca's personal and professional self-development hinged on coming to terms with her need to charge a viable fee and to invest resources in promoting her business.

When Bianca first set up in practice, she did not have a lot of money to spend on advertising and, therefore, could only afford small advertisements in the classified section of her local newspaper under the general heading of "Health". Obviously, such advertisements did not produce a sufficient number of clients to keep the wolf from Bianca's door. At the time, Bianca did not understand the need to consider advertising for her practice as an investment. If Bianca was not seen to be there, then, no-one could ring for an appointment. Hence, Bianca's nagging worry was wrapped up in her motivation not to promote herself adequately.

Similarly, Bianca could not bring herself to charge a realistic fee and she justified her actions by telling herself that she was inexperienced, that she was helping people and that, therefore, she should only charge a very little. The breakthrough for Bianca came when a colleague gave her a stern lecture. Bianca's colleague told her, in no uncertain terms, that therapy was the best thing that her client would ever do for herself in her whole life and it was, consequently, highly appropriate for her to charge a decent fee. When Bianca finally saw the light, she decided to invest in quality advertisements that were on the television page of her local free-bee newspaper on the basis that most people usually look on that page. Bianca's business was, thus, launched with style and success.

With her new-found strength, Bianca eventually cracked the nut when she secured an interview and a phone-in on the radio about a self-help book that she had written. During this radio slot, Bianca had the presence of mind to give out her practice telephone number and, from that point on, she never looked back.

Why would your client choose you?

Will you be astounded when your fish takes the bait and your client arrives? When you lack experience of being a practitioner, you may fear that you will be neglected by your prospective client. Now may be the time for you to examine who you really think you are.

How will you totally believe in yourself?

You may sincerely believe that your client will instantly recognize the experienced professional and merely beat a path to someone else's door. Your lack of self-belief may be particularly relevant if you work in an area where another professional has already established a practice. In these circumstances, you should be prepared for disillusionment. Your prospective client may, for no discernable reason, simply not choose your highly-experienced colleague down the road and you will be left wondering why the magic did not work for someone else.

Your client will choose you not necessarily because she feels you are more experienced, better looking, more accomplished, cheaper or wiser than your colleague. Your client will choose you for her own personal and unique reasons. Your client will be steered towards you inexplicably for reasons of which she may be entirely unaware but her unconscious motivation will be irresistible as well as being mysterious. The phenomenon of transference may, of course, have a strong role to play in the equation for your client. Your client may imagine any number of things about you that will contribute to her final decision about which you may be utterly clueless. You may well remain in total ignorance about your client's motivation to consult you and the best you can do, in these circumstances, can only be to speculate. So both you and your client are likely to come together, as if by magic, and neither of you will have any idea why.

If you are fortunate, your client will have made an informed choice, and will have done the necessary research, in order to select you and only you. In this case, you can probably predict that your client will be right for you and that you will be spot on for her. More often than not, however, your client will select you as her practitioner with very little forethought. If you preen your feathers because your client has chosen you above all others, then, beware the day when you are idle and your colleagues are rushed off their feet. Either way, the best course of action will be for you to detach yourself from any anxiety relating to securing your client and simply leave it all to the fate of the universe. By this means, you will sleep more easily at nights and will not convey your desperation to your prospective client.

Ask yourself ...

Do you really know why your client has chosen you above all others? Did your client like the sound of your voice or the color-scheme of your advertising literature? Would your client have knocked on your door just because you were the nearest practitioner? Would your client have chosen you because you claim to be knowledgeable about a particular disorder that has tormented her for many years? Would your client have researched all the practitioners in your field and, then, made an informed choice? Did your client choose you because she wanted a parent-figure? Might your client have booked a session with you because you remind her of a supportive friend or of Auntie Mabel who was kind to her when she was a child? Did your client select you because you remind her of Uncle Fred who had a bad temper and she, now, wants to get even with him with your help? Does your client come to you because she feels that she can push you around and not really address any of her major health issues? Does your client attend your clinic because she imagines that you are helpful, understanding, caring, professional and competent? Does your client choose to see you because you are young and inexperienced and she wants to help you out? Does your client consider that you are mature and wise and does she sincerely believe that you alone will have all the answers? Did your client learn of your previous successes and could she, now, be curious to find out more because she truly feels that you will be the only one to ever listen? Does your client consider that she has seen so many people who cannot help her and she, now, wants you to confirm her belief that she must be incurable and, at the same time, to prove that you are a complete failure? Does your client, in fact, not really have even the remotest notion about why she has selected you and why she may be attending your practice?

Let's look at it another way – I'll wear a red carnation

When you have a pen-friend, you might get to know each other very well. Perhaps you correspond regularly by letter, by email or by bush telegraph? At first, you may have been tentative in your correspondence with your new-found friend. You may have played it safe and kept the conversation light and jovial. You stick to facts but you conceal the unexpurgated truth about yourself just in case your pal should get scared, run away and, then, leave you with a big hole in your life. After a while, both you and your friend become more adventurous. You tell her a few secrets and your comrade tells you a few too. In no time at all, you are revealing all your secrets and your innermost thoughts to this virtual stranger. It might be as if the sheer anonymity of the blank sheet of paper, or the empty screen, will prompt you to be yourself, safe in the knowledge that your thoughts will be received without judgment or criticism by a close confidant.

To your sheer delight, your friend finally suggests that you might meet for a bite and a chat. Far from being reticent, you agree to the rendezvous with all eagerness. At last, you will be meeting the love of your life, your trusted comrade and your soul-mate. You sweep all minor inhibitions aside and you cannot wait for the day to arrive. Then terror strikes! Perhaps you will get the date or the meeting-time wrong? What if you arrange to meet by the clock-tower but your friend does not turn up? What if you stand on one side of the clock-tower while your pen-pal waits patiently on the other? What if you do not recognize each other, despite having exchanged photographs? The horrors of going to all that effort for nothing loom large in your imagination. Your wise kindred-spirit comes up with the brilliant suggestion of wearing a red carnation while you carry a copy of a magazine dispensing advice about alternative medicine. The rescue-remedy has been found and, now, you can travel to your destination in comfort and in the happy expectation of a successful union.

At the newsstand, however, the magazine has sold out on the appointed day and this causes you instant panic. But, undaunted, you continue your journey, remembering that your associate will still be wearing that essential red carnation, and, thus, serenity returns to you once more. Unbeknown to you, however, your buddy has a woolly memory and, so, she forgets entirely about the joke of the red carnation. When you arrive at the designated clock-tower, nonetheless, you magically and instantly recognize your chum by her welcoming smile and her aura of pleasurable anticipation. Perhaps neither of you actually needed those illusive and errant props? You rejoice in the meeting, perhaps, not even giving a second thought to the way in which you instantly, and without hesitation, established rapport? Maybe that red carnation was superfluous to requirements because you really knew the person whom you were meeting that day? The coming together of kin-

dred-souls can, indeed, be a strange and unfathomable phenomenon. Will you really need the red carnation in your buttonhole?

Let's take an example – Regan's story

Regan was virtually penniless when she started her spiritual psychotherapy practice. Regan lived in the posh part of a council estate and the car that stood outside her door was dilapidated to say the very least. Regan worried about her environment but had no choice but to work from home because she could not afford to rent accommodation elsewhere.

When Regan started to focus on establishing her business, and her clients came rolling in, she came to the conclusion that image and presentation were obviously not everything. Regan's client appeared to be oblivious of her surroundings or just chose to ignore the unfashionable part of town in which she worked. It soon dawned on Regan that she had a special quality to which her client was attracted. Once a client had met Regan, and had received the appropriate treatment, the environs became unimportant. Moreover, the ambiance and the healing received by Regan's client was of far greater value to her than the materialistic façade. Regan, therefore, began to believe in herself much more and to have confidence in her work. With her new-found self-assurance, Regan began to flourish and to worry less. When her bank balance improved, of course, Regan was able to find a more suitable venue for her residence and her practice. Regan's upward spiral towards success had, thus, manifested.

What would your stage-fright feel like?

What will jumping off a cliff-edge feel like for you with your client? Before you open your doors as an all-singing-all-dancing practitioner, you will need to foresee the pitfalls and, then, to remove any obstacles to launching and running your business.

How will your inner demons be doing?

Before you ever see your dreaded first client, your innermost demons may begin to rear their ugly heads menacingly. Your unfriendly dragons may well have been dormant to date, if you have been lucky, but, now, as you are just about to jump, there will be no putting off the evil day when they arise dramatically from beneath the surface of your mind.

You may, of course, think that you will be prepared for your first onslaught of clients. You will, undoubtedly, have planned and rehearsed every word that you propose to say to your client and, perhaps, every question that you intend to pose. You may, also, have consulted a wise mentor in order to secure a direction for your client's first session. You may, possibly, have read many books related your client's case and have tenaciously swatted up on the ins and outs of her particular disorder. But, as the hour approaches, the demons will loom larger and some may even get very close and snugly. Worry and sleepless nights could, now, become the norm for you.

Ask yourself . . .

Do you fear that, possibly, your client might not arrive for her scheduled appointment? Do you secretly hope that your very first client will just forget to turn up? Are you petrified that your first client will suffer from a disorder that you have not studied at training college? Maybe your client will know more than you do about therapeutic intervention? Perchance your client will be super-intelligent or will be very worldly-wise? Perhaps your client will intuitively be able to detect that you are a sheer beginner? Maybe your client will instantly recognize that you are a nervous novice and simply walk out? Perhaps your client will expect you to be an utter genius? Maybe your client will insist that you predict her rate of recovery and the length of time that it will take her to get better? Perchance your client will turn out to be a fellow-practitioner who may be more experienced at your game than you are?

Let's look at it another way – Love at first sight

Can you remember when you met your first love? Can you recall the eyelash-fluttering and the uncontrollable blushes? Can you still feel the thrill when the object of your desires, at last, asked you to or agreed to take a walk in the park and to share an ice cream? Can you remember buying a new garment to wear and taking 3 hours to get ready for the date? Do you still quake at the thought of the butterflies and the collie-wobbles? Can you recall those sleepless nights beforehand and having no appetite for lunch? Was the anticipation of sheer ecstasy as the clock ticked on too much to endure for one so young and innocent?

Of course, you can recall your first kiss and your first fumble. Your first introduction to sexual maturity will be something that you will never forget.

When that pair of delicious lips intrepidly touched yours for the first time, did you consider, for a moment, that it might have been the first time for your partner, too. And would you have cared anyway? The excitement, the climax and the elation of that first kiss might have been so all-consuming that you would have been transported to seventh heaven and have really not returned for many days. Maybe your partner had the same experience? Who knows? But will you ever be the same again? What do you think about the law of attraction?

Let's take an example – Beatrice's story

Beatrice knew that, when starting out in practice as a hypnotherapist, she was her own worst enemy. Beatrice's fears were looming large about the fact that she would create her own disasters when her client knocked on the door. Beatrice, for example, had always worried about the possibility of her client falling asleep after which she would not be able to awaken her. This theme ran through Beatrice's mind when on her training course and, still, lingered even when she first began to practice.

Eventually, one of Beatrice's clients did actually fall fast asleep. The self-fulfilling prophecy had manifested. Tactic one was for Beatrice to suggest to her client that she arouse herself but this was to no avail. In desperation, Beatrice decided to awaken her client by gentle, physical persuasion in order to restore her to full consciousness. It transpired, then, that Beatrice's client was simply exhausted and what she desperately required was to obtain some much-needed rest. Moreover, it appeared that Beatrice's client had, also, fallen asleep in order to avoid addressing some of her sensitive issues. In a sense, Beatrice's client had, in fact, been surprised at the deeply investigative nature of her therapy and, thus, her mind had found a convenient means of delaying cathartic revelation by actually switching off. Hypnotherapy had, thus, given Beatrice's client much more than she had originally bargained for. After this incident, however, Beatrice no longer harbored her greatest fear because she had experienced her demon in the flesh. Beatrice, of course, also, learned to accept that, on given occasions, her client might take a while to come out of her relaxed state during hypnotherapy but that this was not really any real cause for concern.

What would your disaster-scenario feel like?

What will true hell really feel like for you with your client? At some point in your professional life, be assured of the fact that you will make an error. The only deciding factor will be dictated by the way in which you can cope with this uncalled for disaster.

How will you court inevitable disaster?

It may help you to imagine your worst-case scenario as a means of extinguishing your real fears about the end of the world with your client. You may need to begin by recalling all those times in your life when you had to face your demons. Get used to the fact that your gremlins may still be lingering inside ready to pounce at any second. The demon of disaster will, of course, strike with your client when you least expect it. When the demon of disaster does strikes, moreover, it may feel as if your client has complete control of your destiny and that she knows precisely what you might be thinking.

At this point, behold the fiend in front of you. Introduce yourself and get to know this unwanted creature. Your demon may look gruesome or daunting. Your dragon may hold a whip or a club with which to beat you mercilessly. Your devil may have a menacing look or a slimy smirk. Your fierce giant may tower above you with an air of authority and supremacy. The demon of disaster, however, will definitely be the one to be conquered. Find a way of wiping that supercilious grin off your demon's face. See your tormentor crumbling at your command. Watch your demon cowering and quaking in your presence. Imagine your giant shriveling and shrinking at only one glance from you. Watch your evil spirit getting smaller and smaller down to the level of total insignificance. And, when your gremlin gets to the size of a worm, then, merely step on this trifling detail and watch it crumble beneath your feet. Reduce your demon to a non-entity, soon to be forgotten as not worth even a single thought. Finally, know that if ever your demon should even consider returning to plague you, then, it can be given a much stronger and repeated dose of your treatment.

Ask yourself . . .

Can you vividly imagine total disaster striking your practice? Can you visualize what it would be like if your world caved in? Perhaps you can remember being very small and living in that world of powerful giants? Can you envisage what it would be like to be the victim of a volcanic eruption? Can you imagine being totally out of control, utterly abandoned and bereft? Can you imagine being lost, desperate, powerless and helpless? When was that time in your life when the world was such a terrifying and confusing place for one so young and tiny? Can you imagine what your demon looks like and what it might be saying to you? Can you successfully and regularly banish your demon of disaster?

Let's take an example – Desdemona's story

When Desdemona qualified as a rebirthing practitioner, she was gushing with enthusiasm and with high hopes about launching her therapeutic practice. Desdemona was, thus, expecting to see shed-loads of clients and to have a flourishing business in no time at all. Burning with eagerness, Desdemona took out her first advertisement for her would-be clients. Desdemona, then, waited anxiously for the telephone to ring but, however, the anticipated explosion did not occur.

Desdemona soon realized that she was not only brimming with enthusiasm but also with desperation. When a prospective client telephoned, Desdemona could not contain herself and her excitement. Several clients rang to ask a few questions but did not book. Others came for a free consultation but, still, did not book. The desperation stakes were getting high for Desdemona. Finally, Desdemona realized that her keenness was turning to a form of nervousness that her prospective client could probably detect. When this realization dawned, Desdemona, then, let go of her longing and, hey presto, the tide turned. Desdemona had, therefore, surmounted an important learning-curve in that she had discovered how to cool down when talking to her prospective client.

Desdemona, also, learned how to listen and how to respond appropriately to her enquirer's needs. Desdemona, moreover, began to appreciate that she did not need to attempt to convince her prospective client of her prowess as a practitioner. Desdemona discovered that any serious enquirer would not be, at all, interested in her long string of exemplary qualifications and her impressive accomplishments. Desdemona, therefore, learned how to play the practitioner's game with subtlety. Desdemona soon, then, began to obtain bookings and to retain her clients and she, now, charges for her initial consultation. Desdemona's business and her peace of mind have, thus, benefited from her early experiences in the world of being a professional practitioner as well as being an effective publicity agent.

11 HOW WOULD YOU COMPILE YOUR PUBLICITY BROCHURE?

Why would you need a promotional brochure?

Will you really be ready to make a statement to the world and to your client? The purpose of your publicity brochure will be for you to attract your prospective client and to answer the kind of questions that she may have about you and your practice.

Will you survive without a publicity vehicle?

The mainstay of any practitioner's publicity material will usually be a personalized brochure and this vehicle will, almost certainly, be your starting point in terms of your relationship with the public. You may be able to bypass business cards, letterheads, compliments slips and handout leaflets but it may be that your business cannot exist without a brochure of some kind in order to advertise your services.

Often the compilation of your publicity brochure will be your first step on the road towards launching your business. Failure to produce your personal brochure may, also, be evidence of the fact that you do not really want to get started. If you find yourself lagging behind in terms of compiling your brochure and, therefore, launching your business, then, listen carefully to your inner voice. Do not, of course, take that first step until you are entirely sure that you will want to go there. If you are determined to tread the practitioner's path, then, compiling your brochure may, in fact, be a daunting task but one that you, as a resolute pioneer, will find a way of overcoming.

Ask yourself . . .

Can you see the need to publicize yourself by compiling a publicity vehicle in the guise of a brochure? Do you feel fired up with enthusiasm for compiling your brochure that you can proudly show to the world? Do you consider that producing your brochure will be a statement that you are not yet ready to make? Can you really make do with some literature provided by your professional body? Could compiling your brochure be something that you will keep pushing to the foot of your personal agenda? Are you putting off the evil day with regard to creating your brochure because you really do not want to become a working professional? Do you feel that you do not need any publicity material because you already have a viable market for your services? Do you need more time in order to consolidate your learning before you can launch your practice?

How would you write the text for your brochure?

Will you be able to tell it like it is about yourself to your client? Producing your promotional brochure may not be a task that you can defer indefinitely once you have decided that you would need one. Getting starting on compiling your brochure will usually be evidence of your personal commitment to launching your business both physically and mentally. So, once you are geared up and ready to go, the sooner you get started on this, perhaps, tedious administrative task the better.

How will you put your brochure text together?

Writing your brochure may seem a thoroughly awesome task especially if writing happens not to be your forte but, in fact, all you may really need to do will be to provide some information about yourself and your practice. You will not be required to attempt to transform yourself into a creative copywriter. If the task of producing your brochure really does seem beyond your capabilities, however, then, simply ask someone else to do it for you. Always, of course, ensure that, in these circumstances, you will have the overall control and the final decision on the content and the wording. A halfway house may be to filch the wording wholesale from another friendly practitioner, although this route should really only be used as a short-term measure and may not give you the much-needed satisfaction of putting your own stamp on it.

Your brochure should ideally be a unique and personal statement about you and it should be written from the heart. Writing your brochure should not, therefore, be a five-minute, Friday afternoon job and it will, almost inevitably, need to be revised numerous times before you can circulate it worldwide with pride. Compiling your publicity brochure might, of necessity, be a time-consuming exercise because it will be the world's introduction to you as a professional. The good news will be that, once you have devised the text for your brochure, you can, then, easily transpose this wording to a website, to a handout leaflet or to any other form of advertising material that you may care to generate.

Before starting to compile your brochure, you should borrow as many brochures as you can from other practitioners, especially those in your own particular field. Note the different styles of writing and the various approaches to the task of painting the picture that others will have employed. Reading the material of others should stimulate your ideas and you could, possibly, even pinch a few carefully-chosen phrases and, then, disguise them as your own invention. If your professional body or your former training establishment publishes literature, then, this too can be an excellent source of reference. You may find that your professional association, for instance, will have devised the definitive wording for describing your therapeutic practice and there will, therefore, be no need for you to reinvent the wheel.

Prior to going to press, it may be a good ploy for you to seek the opinion of several other practitioners both in your own field and in other therapeutic disciplines. This insurance policy can, at least, minimize the risk of ambiguities, factual errors, design-faults, irrelevance, nonsense, omissions and textual inaccuracies. Even after worldwide circulation, you may still need to update your brochure's text frequently and regularly for, at least, the first few months after launching your practice. You may, thereafter, wish to update your brochure at regular intervals in order to reflect your professional growth. Remember that your publicity brochure will be a personal statement about you and you are likely to be constantly changing and spiritually evolving.

Ask yourself . . .

Do you dread the fact that you will need to compile your brochure and do you feel stuck for ideas? Can you find a means of manifesting inspiration about what to include in your brochure by reading what others might have to say? Can you have a brainstorming session with your own creative imagination? What would your personal mission statement about yourself and your future business say in a nutshell? Can you capture the essence of what you feel about your practice in words? What does your professional association or your training body have to say about your therapeutic discipline? Can you obtain a copy of a brochure from a known colleague or a trusted mentor? Can you write your brochure and, then, show it to others who will be able to appraise its wording and its design and, then, give you some constructive criticism?

How would you produce copies of your brochure?

Will you be able to assess the most cost-effective route towards promoting yourself to your client? Much thought may need to be devoted to the way in which you will structure and will reproduce your advertising brochure before you even start to put pen to paper.

Will you be able to visualize your finished product?

A typical alternative practitioner's brochure will usually consist of one sheet of A4-sized paper folded into three equal portions. A more expensive version of this idea would be to use one or more sheets of A4-sized paper folded in two, perhaps, with a thicker front cover.

If you have access to a computer, this may be your salvation when producing your brochure. Not only will you be able to write and to refine your text numerous times but you will, also, be able to do the typesetting yourself and this may save you some dosh. If you do not have ready access to a computer, then, life may be considerably more difficult until you can find a tame friend who can help you, if only to type the text that you might later give to a printer. The advantage of using a computer will be the flexibility and the cost-saving, especially if you only intend to generate relatively small quantities of your final product. Once completed, your brochure can, then, be printed on reasonably plain paper from your local stationery store. You may, also, elect to purchase some specialist brochure paper or some thin card that has been pre-printed and/or pre-folded for that extra touch of class.

It will, of course, be perfectly possible for you to give the entire task to a printer who will produce a professional-looking brochure but this route will only make economic sense if you intend to print your brochure in bulk. You might, however, be able to save on typesetting costs by compiling your brochure on your own computer and, then, shipping the computer file to the typesetter. Be aware, of course, that if you print, say, 500 or 5000 brochures, and, then, wish to change your mind completely about what you have said, you could regret it financially. In the early days of establishing your business, therefore, the posh printing route may be a game of Russian-roulette for you.

Ask yourself . . .

Have you considered the finer details of your brochure's layout and its reproduction? Can you find the simplest yet the most cost-effective route for producing your personal brochure that will, also, offer flexibility? Does your brochure portray the right publicity image for you? Does your brochure need to be elaborate or to be atmospheric? Does your brochure need a professional designer's skill? Should your brochure appear to be businesslike and professional yet still harness the personal touch? Will you need to beg, steal or borrow a computer for the task of producing the wording for your brochure? Have you researched the type and the quality of paper or card on to which you could print your computer text? Are you clear, in your mind, about the way in which the text should be laid out and formatted? Can you check out the cost and the quality of producing your brochure with your local printer?

How would you know what information to convey?

What will your prospective client need to hear from you? Because your publicity brochure may be your potential client's first and only introduction to you as a working professional, you will need to carefully vet every word that you say.

Will you predict the psyche of your target audience?

Remember to get into your prospective client's mind in order to predict what she will want to know before making a positive decision to book a session with you. The key ingredient of your brochure should be to answer all your prospective client's questions and to convey encouragement and reassurance. Your client will need to know what your therapeutic practice can offer and what it will entail for her. Your brochure should, therefore, portray you with an aura of professionalism, coupled with a warm and welcoming touch. In essence, your brochure should give a description of your therapeutic methodology and what you will have to offer to your prospective client. Your voice, as an individual, should come through strongly so that your prospective client can be assured that there will be a real-live person behind the therapeutic mask.

Ask yourself . . .

Will your client want you to allay any misconceptions about your therapeutic practice? Would your client need some encouragement before taking the final plunge? Will your client require some reassurance that she will be getting a treatment suitable for her recovery needs? Might your client wish to know what your therapy entails in some detail? Could your client be reticent about exploring alternative methods of treatment? Will your client need you to confirm that you are a consummate professional in your field? Might your client be anxious about certain key aspects of your therapeutic practice because she may be facing her deepest fears and have a life-threatening condition? Will your client have difficulty in understanding the concept of therapeutic treatment that can only really be understood by first-hand experience? Would you be able to beckon your client to consult you without twisting her arm?

Which writing style would you adopt?

Will you be able to hit the happy medium between being red hot and ice cold with your client? You should choose a consistent writing style for your brochure and, indeed, for all your publicity material, that should be in keeping with the kind of therapeutic services that you will be offering to your client.

Will you be formal and friendly simultaneously?

Getting it right will mean choosing a writing style that will suit your unique personality, will cater for your personal preferences and will be appropriate for your profession. There can be no right and no wrong answers to this issue for you. It will simply be a case of going with your gut instincts and, then, sticking to your guns until you decide to change horses. But first consider the various options you might have before even turning on the computer and, then, use these decisions as your starting point.

You will need to choose whether a formal and, perhaps, slightly impersonal style will be appropriate for your practice or whether you will need to adopt a friendly and even chatty approach. An informal approach would employ the second person singular (addressing your client as "you") in order to create the impression that you are providing a personal service for your client. A formal style would employ the third person singular (referring to your client as "the client") as a means of conveying an atmosphere of unbiased opinion in order to demonstrate a clinical approach. Ideally, a middle-of-the-road course will usually be the best but this will be a choice that you alone must make. Certainly the personal touch will normally be a good idea when delivering a personal service. Whichever course you intend to take, however, do not do a hard-selling job or appear to be too desperate.

Ask yourself . . .

Will a formal style, written in the third person singular, be suitable for you as a serious clinical professional? Will an informal approach, written in the second person singular, be in keeping with the welcoming service that you intend to offer to your client? Will a hands-on approach in which you convey personal information about your own healing experiences be appropriate? Are you offering an in-depth, psychologically-oriented therapy that might demand a detached and formal style? Are you offering a service that will require you to put your client at ease and, therefore, should be in keeping with a relaxed writing style? Do you wish to portray yourself as an open-house practitioner who will accept all comers? Do you wish to be selective in terms of your clients and, thus, not tolerate any time-wasters? Do you desire to show that you are businesslike and in an officially-recognized profession? Will your chosen writing style scream of hard-sell tactics? Can you write your brochure with a judicial mixture of confidence, compassion, conviction, love, passion and sincerity?

What personal information would you convey?

Will you really choose to reveal all about yourself to your client? The basic information that you will need to include in your brochure should cover who you are, what you do and the way in which you could help your prospective client. Your future client will, of course, want to know something about you, as a person, and her understandable curiosity should, in some manner, be adequately satisfied by you.

What will your client need to know about you?

When adding that personal touch to your brochure, you may wish to consider very carefully the way in which you will promote yourself as an individual. An adequate amount of personal information can portray you as a praiseworthy human being but too much detail could expose you in the wrong light. Remember that it will be your client who comes to you to be listened to and not the other way around.

Your name, your contact details and your practice location should obviously be prominently displayed in order to make it easy for your client to contact you. Your client may wish to have an initial discussion with you, or to book an appointment without delay, when the time might be exactly right for her. If your contact details are in the small print, this may be enough to dissuade your client from contacting you, particularly, if she has been teetering on the brink of indecision. If your contact information, on the other hand, has been set in headline-sized type, this may, also, be off-putting to your client who may assume that you wish to seek the limelight.

It may be wise for you to state your qualifications in terms of your basic professional training, together with any advanced or any additional training that you might have undertaken. In a well-known and/or a legally-regulated profession, your prospective client may require the assurance that you do, in fact, possess the official and the appropriate qualifications. In most cases, your qualifications will mean virtually nothing to your prospective client but a note of these will, at least, give her some indication that you are a bona fide practitioner and will, hopefully, look impressive anyway. When it comes to talking about your professional qualifications, your client should be reassured that you are equipped to do the job and that she will be in the care of a skilled expert. It may, moreover, be beneficial for you to state any specialist qualifications or any special interests that you may have acquired in connection with your practice methodology.

You may wish to include information about any professional body of which you are a member, together with a statement verifying that you are covered by professional insurance and by public liability insurance, as appropriate. You may, furthermore, elect to include the logo of your professional body within your literature as your signature of bona fide practice.

What will be your terms and conditions of practice?

Always state clearly any terms and conditions that will apply to your client when she attends your practice. You may wish to include your pricing structure, the time-length of your sessions and the rules that would pertain to any cancellations or any non-attendance. If you work only on specific days of the week, or only during certain times, it may be advantageous for you to include this information in order to forewarn your prospective client who may feel that she can blithely consult you on Sunday afternoon at teatime. You may, however, not wish to include specific details of the fees that you charge, particularly, if you are having a couple of thousand brochures printed that will last you several years during which time your prices will increase. This obstacle can usually be overcome by inviting your prospective client to telephone you for more information or you could simply produce a separate price list for inclusion with your brochure.

Will you wish to include a personal photograph?

If you can afford it, you could include a photograph of yourself as a means of introducing yourself to your client. Do, of course, ensure that your picture will be large enough and be clear enough for you to be easily recognized by your prospective client. Remember to portray yourself as a caring, a sincere and an utterly professional practitioner. Do not make the mistake of using a tatty, unflattering mugshot taken at the local, quick-and-easy passport machine. Moreover, do not use some glamour shot that was taken in the days when you were young and beautiful and were pursuing a career in the film industry. It would be wise to ask several other practitioners for their opinion of your photograph before you even contemplate including it in your publicity material. Your photograph should, at least, have a professional look about it, despite the fact that you may not elect to employ a professional photographer in order to do the job for you.

What will be your personal mission statement?

It will usually be sensible for you to include a section in your brochure that will give a personal statement about your commitment to your work. Remember that your mission statement will be a personal proclamation about your beliefs that should assist your prospective client to relate to you as a professional and caring individual. Your personal statement can include information about the therapy that you offer, your qualifications, any legal or regulatory requirements, any specializations, any special therapeutic interests, where you trained, when you first qualified, why you trained, any particular special achievements and, if appropriate, some brief personal details.

Let's take an example – A craniosacral therapist

X uses gentle, non-invasive touch and subtle treatment skills without manipulation to both identify and treat distress and disorder held in the body. X can, also, draw from a background of holistic counseling with methods ranging from nutrition to vibrational healing.

Let's take an example – An infant massage instructor

X is a mother of two, qualified Massage Therapist and Infant Massage Instructor. She is, also, trained as a Doula (childbirth companion). X brings her own unique approach to facilitating classes and teaching massage, including her experience of yoga, breathing techniques, meditation, visualization and singing.

Let's take an example – A medical herbalist

I gained a BSc (Hons) in Herbal Medicine at Middlesex University. I furthered my interest in plant medicine by qualifying in aromatherapy and massage. I am a member of the International Federation of Professional Aromatherapists (IFPA) and the National Institute of Medical Herbalists (NIMH). I use where possible organic or biodynamic herbs from suppliers committed to quality and environmentally-friendly growing and production methods. I do not use plants that are endangered or taken from fragile resources. All medicines are of plant origin and are free from animal products.

Let's take an example – A reflexologist

X has been in natural healing for some years. Her approach to the feet through Universal Reflexology is all encompassing of the physical, mental and emotional bodies. X became the founder, principal and tutor of her own school of complementary therapy and currently runs a busy practice. All of her work has been focused on empowerment of the individual. Reflexology enforces the belief that disease and illness is psychosomatic and stress-related. The body is naturally healthy and it is only unnatural thoughts, fears and emotions that upset its natural equilibrium. Emotions are immediately reflected in the physical body as ease or disease. Reflexology can treat an extensive range of complaints as well as having a profound effect on the management of day to day living. X has a special interest in fertility, pregnancy and childbirth.

How would you describe your therapy?

Will you be able to educate your client convincingly? The essence of your publicity brochure will be concerned with what your therapeutic specialty might be all about, generally, and what it will have to offer your prospective client, specifically. An introduction to your therapeutic practice should normally include a description of your particular field of work and should, also, outline what treatment may entail for your client.

What will be the purpose of introducing your therapy?

Your prospective client should be left in no doubt whatsoever about the therapeutic services that you have to offer, the way in which your treatment could help her and, if possible, what the healing process will entail. Because many alternative therapies are almost impossible to explain in words, the purpose of this section of your literature will be to give your client enough information in order to whet her appetite. Your client can, consequently, be induced to take the plunge, safe in the knowledge that she will be in good hands.

In this section of your brochure, you might need to go into specifics if your practice methodology might not be common knowledge. If you practice an ancient method of healing, for example, it may be prudent for you to emphasize this vital point and, simultaneously, to provide your client with an assurance of a proven efficacy that has stood the test of time. If your little-known therapeutic methodology has originated as an offshoot from another practice, then, it might be wise to mention this fact to your client. Moreover, you may wish to state the philosophy that underpins your practice as this may well be the reason why your client will decide to book an appointment with you.

Your starting place, when compiling the text for your practice statement will, probably, be the literature published by your training college or your professional body. For this reason, you may wish to consider the material written by your professional association so that you can utilize the wording while, perhaps, condensing and distilling your own ideas. If you are smart, you can steer a cunning course between not reinventing the wheel, because someone else has put time and thought into describing your therapy, and, simultaneously, putting your own personal spin on the facts. Down this route, you will be in a catch-all, win-win situation.

Ask yourself . . .

Will your client wish to know whether you are conducting a therapy with eastern or western origins? Will your client need to be reassured that your therapy will be one that has a proven track-record and has stood the test of time? Might your client wish to appreciate the subtle mechanics of your practice? Might your client desire to know the philosophy behind the way in which your therapy can work for her? Will your client need to grasp the fact that you are offering an energetic or a vibrational methodology? Should your client be told whether you are practicing a treatment in which supplements are prescribed that might cost extra money? Will your client want to be assured that your therapy will be the best possible route that she can take on her road to recovery?

Let's take an example – Acupuncture

Acupuncture has a practice history extending over 2000 years. It works by stimulating points of different areas of the body. Such stimulation aims to direct the body, as a whole, into a state of balance. Chinese Medicine believes health is achieved, and maintained, when our bodies are balanced and in harmony.

Let's take an example – Colonic hydrotherapy

Colonic hydrotherapy is a safe and effective method of removing waste, encrusted matter, mucus, gas, toxins and parasites from the large intestine, using warm, filtered water. All equipment is sterilized using hospital-approved solutions. The water is filtered and administered via a gravitational system, i.e. a slow flow, so there is no excess pressure on the bowel. Colonic hydrotherapy is not habit forming and can improve the muscle tone of the bowel. The use of laxatives is, however, habit forming and can make the bowel become lazy.

Let's take an example – Flower and gem essences

Flower and gem essences are liquid plant or gem preparations which carry a unique message of healing from the specific flower or gem. They recognize a relationship between our physical body and the spiritual, mental and emotional aspects of wellness. Over time they can help to clear trauma from cellular memory and our energy field, resulting in enhanced physical, emotional and psychological wellbeing. Flower and gem essences are catalysts for change and stimulate the ability to respond to and take responsibility for life challenges.

Let's take an example – Homeopathy

For two hundred years, homeopathy as been recognized as a uniquely effective method of healing. It works by stimulating the body's natural

287

healing powers through small doses of remedies that actually match the symptoms shown; remedies made from plants, minerals and even poisons. Homeopathy treats not merely the symptoms, the effects of illness or disease, but helps deal with their basic causes. As the immune system does the curative work, it is crucial that the whole person, and not just the diseased part, is treated. The whole person is more than a collection of separate, physical organs.

What would be the scope of your therapy?

Will you ever be able to cover all the bases with your client? Your prospective client may wish to know the way in which she can specifically benefit from your branch of alternative practice. Your client may, in fact, need to identify precisely whether the condition from which she has been suffering can be addressed by your therapy. You may, therefore, find it useful to provide a list of those conditions that your therapeutic methodology can be used to treat and those, if any, for which it cannot claim to provide any assistance.

What will you say about your therapy?

Do not ever make any exaggerated claims about what you can treat and do not even attempt to imply that you can cure anything. If necessary, emphasize that it will be your client's responsibility to affect a result and that you can only merely assist in the process.

Your training college or your professional association may, in some instances, provide some guidelines as to, say, a recommended number of sessions or any general treatment outcomes. In these circumstances, you may elect to include such information in your brochure. Be aware, of course, that any recommendations that you do quote to your client will be your responsibility and not that of another authority. Without knowing anything about your client in advance, of course, it could be a dangerous game to stipulate rigidly the way in which she could be treated. The old adage of "how long is a piece of string?" will, essentially, be the only guarantee that you can provide in the field of remedial, curative therapy in terms of treatment-length. It may, also, be wise to be mindful of the fact that recovery will simply be a notion in your client's mind and, perhaps, an improvement may only be the ultimate possibility for her. As an alternative practitioner, of course, it may be advantageous for you to develop the art of generalization in order to safeguard your position with your client.

Ask yourself . . .

Will your client need to know what your therapy can and cannot achieve? Will your client be interested to know that your therapy can be used in a preventative capacity as well as being a curative methodology? Will your client need to find out whether she must make an expensive long-term commitment to your therapy? Might you regret it later if you are too pedantic about what you claim in terms of treatment outcomes for your client? Will your client be anxious to know how soon she may expect any change in her condition? Will your client want to learn about whether your therapy can help with her depression, her backache, her eating-disorder, her hormonal imbalance, her skin-rash or her forgetfulness?

Let's take an example – The Alexander technique

The Technique improves balance, co-ordination and poise; and leads to greater control. It is used at every level of sport and the arts to enhance performance and prevent injury. John McEnroe, Yehudi Menuhin and Judi Dench are amongst many famous users of the Technique. Alexander Technique lessons gradually improve your confidence and sense of wellbeing and can form a basis for learning any new skill.

Let's take an example – Indian head massage

Indian head massage is a traditional treatment, used by Indian women for over 1000 years. It is most effective for alleviating stress and tension. Working on the upper back, shoulders, neck and head, the massage gently but firmly releases any stress or tension from these areas. This part of the treatment is a dry massage, directly on the skin. The massage continues on the scalp, using a specific blend of oils, which is said to promote hair growth, although no promises are given! This again releases any tension, and gives a feeling of wellbeing. This is followed by massage of the face, bringing further relaxation. The session finishes with healing, to rebalance the whole body.

Let's take an example – McTimoney chiropractic

The gentle nature of the McTimoney chiropractic technique makes it especially suitable for people of all ages including young, pregnant women and the elderly. Are you suffering from any of the following conditions: back, neck and shoulder pain; pain, discomfort and stiffness in joints and bones; migraine and tension headaches; muscular aches and pains; sciatica; whiplash injury, sport injuries? McTimoney chiropractic may improve any of the above.

Let's take an example – Rebirthing

Rebirthing has many, many benefits because it affects all areas of your life – the mind being behind everything we create or don't create in our lives. It particularly helps with the following: it opens up and frees your breath; it heals birth and childhood patterns which may well be affecting your life; it lifts you out of anxiety and depression; it frees up your emotions; it helps you feel good about your sexuality and resolves any relationship issues/blocks you may have; it gives you vastly improved confidence and the ability to communicate easily, without blame; it helps you feel connected and at one and generally it will lead you to high self-esteem and, very important, healing 'the child within'. It can, also, help you find your life purpose – because we all have one – and what's more: be successful in achieving this.

What would be your practice methodology?

How will you do your thing with your client in the therapeutic context? Often your client will be interested or, perhaps, concerned to know what a typical therapeutic session will entail. It could be that your client may know nothing of the methodology that you will employ but may want to be enlightened. Alternatively, your client may simply be curious about what to expect and her curiosity should, of course, be satisfied.

Will you allay your client's misgivings?

Your job in compiling your publicity brochure will be to explain your therapeutic methodology as succinctly as possible to your prospective client. Your client may, in fact, have experienced your branch of therapeutic practice previously but she may still need to know what to expect from you and whether your practice might differ, in any way, from her past experience. Your client may, of course, be quite apprehensive about undertaking a treatment of which she, currently, remains in ignorance. Your client may, also, be in total disbelief about the way in which some off-the-wall alternative therapy could, possibly, help her to overcome her disorder. Your client, in whatever her circumstances, will have the right to know what to expect from your methodology but her curiosity will be a sign that, at least, she could be tempted.

Ask yourself . . .

Will your client be concerned to establish whether you personally have specific experience of her particular condition? Will your client be anxious to know whether she will need to undress, to remain fully clothed or to wear any special garments? Might your client be concerned to know whether she will need to change her diet radically or whether she will be asked to take any horrid-tasting medicine? Will your client need to know whether you will encourage her to delve into her childhood or to get in contact with her emotional life? Will your client be concerned about whether you will touch her or will inflict any pain? Might your client endeavor to discover whether she needs to believe in the angelic realm or in the life hereafter? Will your client need to know whether she should have a good imagination or if she should be able to relax well? Would your client have been falsely indoctrinated by the media and have gained some idiotic misconceptions about your therapeutic practice? Will your client have had a rather unpleasant introduction to your therapy from another practitioner?

Let's take an example – The Bowen technique

The practitioner uses thumbs and fingers on precise points on the body making rolling-type movements which aim to stimulate energy into the muscles and soft tissue. During the treatment, the therapist will leave the room for short periods, allowing the client to rest while the body processes the moves that have been performed. The Bowen Technique encourages realignment of the body; there is no manipulation of hard tissue and no force is used or needed. Treatment at regular intervals can help manage stress and encourage health maintenance.

Let's take an example – Hypnotherapy

Hypnosis is an entirely natural occurrence. It is an extremely pleasant and relaxing trance state, and everybody has the ability to enter this state. People spontaneously enter trance states on a daily basis as they watch TV, read books, use computers, or even spend time just thinking or day dreaming. Hypnosis is often referred to as conscious hypnosis since the person in hypnosis is not asleep. Frequently, as their senses become heightened in trance, they are more aware than usual of what is taking place, and can, also, converse quite easily while hypnotized.

Let's take an example – Nutritional therapy

To be healthy we need to provide the body with the building blocks to do the job. Illness and unpleasant symptoms are often simply due to deficiencies in some essential elements. We truly are what we eat! At your consultation we will work through your history, symptoms and present diet. From this I will be able to assess what the underlying causes are that give you problems. My recommendations will include advice on diet and food supplements, which are carefully calculated to meet your personal requirements through an individual, tailor-made program and I will summarise everything for you in an easy-to-understand written report.

Let's take an example – Shamanic healing

What is Shamanic Healing & Soul Retrieval? Shamanic Healing consists of a varied body of practices performed by the shaman or practitioner to help or heal another person. This is a fundamental principle of shamanism wherever it is practiced. The methods, tools, symbology, and medicines will vary from culture to culture and region to region but primarily the healing is a three-way connection between the client, shaman and the universe or spirit. The shaman acts as the mediator or interpreter for the universal field of consciousness of which we are all a part.

How would you pull all the strings together?

Will you be discreetly selective while telling all to your client? Because your brochure will be a unique personal statement about you and your therapeutic practice, you may need to take stock before finally committing anything concrete to paper.

Will you know what your finished brochure should comprise?

Perhaps you could utilize a checklist in order to decide on the contents of your publicity brochure. In using your checklist, you can be selective about what information you might wish to include and, then, you can decide what will be important for you to personally convey. Although, in practice, you may not wish to include several of the items in your checklist, you may well need to answer these questions personally by way of preparing yourself for the questions that your prospective client may ask you during any preliminary discussion (see Figure 11.1 – *What might your publicity brochure include?*).

Contact details

Your name? Your practice address? Your practice location map or directions? Your practice telephone number? Your direct line telephone number? Your fax number? Your email address? Your website address?

Personal information

Your professional qualification(s)? The date(s) of gaining your qualification(s)? The training body/bodies with whom you have studied? The duration of your training course(s)? Any specialist or advanced training? Any relevant experience? Any specialist interests? Any requirements for continuing professional development? Any testimonials from satisfied clients? Your membership of any professional association(s)? Reference to your professional insurance? Reference to your practice code of ethics? An outline of your own healing journey? Your reasons for becoming a practitioner?

Therapy description

Your therapy's underlying philosophy? Your therapy's relevant history? Your approach to therapeutic practice? Any specialist aims of treatment? Any specialist methodology employed? How could your therapy work for your client? What might a typical session involve? What can your client expect from her therapy? Will your client need to prepare, in any way, for her session? Will your client feel any after-effects from her session? Will you be required to adopt any specific safety procedures? Will there be any published statistics to support the efficacy of your therapy? Have you obtained any feedback from other clients? Can your client obtain further information from your professional body about your therapy?

Therapy scope

How can your client can be assisted? Would your therapy be suitable and appropriate for your client? How can your therapy be effective for your client's disorder? Can your therapy treat any specific symptoms or conditions? Which disorders can your therapy claim to assist? What contraindications should your client appreciate? Is your therapy an alternative to standard medical or surgical practice? Does your therapy complement standard medical or surgical practice? Is your therapy mainly curative, preventative or both? Will your client's initial session be different from any subsequent sessions? Will your client be expected to attend her sessions regularly or at given intervals? Will you suggest or stipulate a given number of sessions for your client? Will you offer one-to-one sessions and/or group therapy?

Terms and conditions

Your working times or periods? Your fee for an initial consultation? Your fee for any follow-up consultations? Will you offer a free introductory consultation? Will you offer any concessionary rates? Will your client need to pay any additional fees for supplements or remedies? Will your client be required to pay your fee in advance or on the day of her session? Will you only accept cash or cheques? Will you have credit card or debit card facilities? Will you offer any home-visits? Will you make any special arrangements for disabled clients? Will you be required to adopt any special procedures in connection with your professional conduct guidelines?

Figure 11.1 – *What might your publicity brochure include?*

If you, also, carefully consider a number of examples of publicity brochures that have been published by established practitioners, you will often be able to appreciate that the essential ingredients have been included and where the personal touch has come through. Utilize any suitable examples produced by others in order to give yourself inspiration about what to include in your publicity brochure and the way in which you could convey the necessary information to your prospective client.

12 HOW WOULD YOU PROMOTE YOURSELF?

How would you plan your promotional campaign?

Will you be going all out for the full media-spotlight when attracting your prospective client? When planning to launch, to expand and/or to maintain your business, careful consideration will need to be given by you about your promotional approach and the nature of your publicity material. Once you start to plan and execute your publicity campaign, you may find that you will acquire the appetite that comes with eating and this will, then, carry you forth.

What will your publicity material comprise?

Many decisions will need to be made by you about your publicity material and your plan of attack. Putting this package together will be a wonderful means of concentrating your mind on the way in which you will approach the world and your prospective client. Leaving this aspect of business life to chance will not be a good move on your part.

Be well equipped in terms of publicity material of which your personal brochure will, undoubtedly, be the prime selling agent. In many cases, once you have compiled your publicity brochure, the wording can be reused again and again in order to produce any other form of written literature that you may require. As well as producing your publicity brochure, other promotional aids could include some business cards, handouts, posters, mailshots, paid advertisements, free press-releases and a website.

When producing any advertising material, you will, again, need to consider whether you will want to adopt a sober and business-like approach or a jazzy and up-market style. You will, therefore, need to ponder what you want your image to be before you finally begin to make your plans and start to plunge into production.

Ask yourself . . .

Can you plan a phased and integrated promotional campaign for yourself? What will you need to put together in terms of your publicity material and where will you start? Have you considered what your public image should be? Will it be sufficient for you just to have a publicity brochure with nothing else in order to support it? Will you need a website, some advertisements, some flyers or some business cards in order to support your campaign? Which cages could you, possibly, rattle in order to get your voice heard? What facilities can your local library offer you for spreading the word? Can you talk to other practitioners in order to get some hints about how to do it? Do you have enough in the piggy-bank to pay for your luxurious promotions? Will you be able to rely on free advertising and on favors from others in order to promote your work?

How will you get your message across?

Once you have finalized your publicity literature, you may, then, need to find a way of easily circulating it in order to put your message across to the millions. Business promotion will, almost certainly, require some creative thinking on your part and usually a reasonable knowledge of your intended market. All ideas will be good grist to the mill when planning your campaign as these thoughts will form a part of your brainstorming exercise. If you are short of ideas, or want to estimate the likely success of any given option, then, networking with other practitioners may be extremely beneficial in helping you to make the appropriate decisions.

A number of tried and tested methods of business promotion have been successfully employed by up-and-running practitioners and all these options should, at least, be considered by you. Find out about any promotional outlets that colleagues in your own field have previously exploited to good effect and combine these with any other bright ideas you might have. The well-tried channels usually embrace giving a talk to likely candidates, wearing out some shoe-leather in circulating your publicity material and creating a website.

Your local library may welcome receiving publicity information from you that can be passed on to any enquirers. A number of professional bodies will offer to keep a list of their members in order to cater for public enquiries. You should ensure, therefore, that you maintain a presence on any such lists, some of which will be web-based for which you may not need to pay any extra cash. You may, also, find that an entry in a web-directory can attract your prospective market.

If you have recently found your vocation in creative copy-writing, perhaps as a result of compiling your publicity brochure, then, penning a scintillating article for your local newspaper or your area magazine can often go a long way towards launching your business for free. Sometimes your local rag will be hungry for interesting and newsworthy articles, possibly, with an eye-catching photograph of yourself. Always ensure, however, that your article has news-value in that it should tackle anything ordinary from a new angle and ideally should present a unique and never-to-be-missed story. Do not, of course, pick a time during a local election or when a tasty bit of scandal has just hit the press. Find a time when the newspaper or the magazine will be more desperate to fill its pages. Perhaps the best course of action would be for you to telephone your local paper and to chat up the features editor who might even be persuaded to come to your practice in order to have a free taster-treatment in exchange for a sizeable article.

Ask yourself . . .

What have other members of your profession done to promote alternative practice in your area? Can you discover some really creative ways of selling your product? Can you capitalize on any previous sales or any marketing experience that you might possess? Can you get some free advice from an expert in marketing and public relations? Can you research your market in order to discover who might already be there?

Can you predict what your potential client will want to hear? What are your copywriting skills like and could you exploit any personal talents that may be lying dormant? Can you scatter copies of your publicity material in some eye-catching places locally?

How would you deliver a promotional talk?

Will you provide a personal touch when you meet your prospective client? One of the cheapest and usually the most effective ways of reaching your potential client will be to volunteer to give a talk to a captive audience. You could, for instance, contact a number of organizations in your local area who meet regularly and who might be hungry for visiting speakers.

How will you secure your audience for a promotional talk?

Giving a promotional talk to a group of prospective clients will be an ideal way of obtaining some publicity and promoting your services for the cost of a few leaflets and the price of the bus fare. You could contact any local societies or associations who are likely to invite visiting speakers, such as women's groups, social groups and local-interest societies. In most cases, your local library may be a veritable Pandora's box of information on this score. These local organizations will provide you with a captive audience all of whom will have been notified, in advance, of your talk and should, therefore, arrive with interest and curiosity.

Often you can pick up a number of your clients from this fruitful source by spending only a few minutes introducing yourself and your practice. This medium will be an opportunity for your prospective client to see you in the flesh, to gain an understanding of your therapeutic practice and to ask any pressing questions. Be prepared, of course, for your talk to be a dead flop as the worst-case scenario. If this sort of disappointment should occur, then, do not take it personally. Sometimes your audience may be interested but no-one will really be in a position to take up the cudgels. Perhaps your audience-members were too old to care, too penniless to be able to afford your fees or came only for the company and the afternoon tea. In this event, merely put it down to experience and regard your talk, on that occasion, as a full dress-rehearsal for the next one.

Ask yourself . . .

Can you weed out the organizations in your area who might be suitable candidates for an informal talk about your practice? Can you find an exciting way of presenting your subject matter while still retaining the personal touch? How do you feel about standing up and giving a talk in front of a small audience? Can you get some help with your stage-fright before you give your talk? Can you give a talk to a number of people as a means of jettisoning your performance nerves? Can you ask other practitioners about their experiences of talking to small audiences?

What will your promotional talk include?

The purpose of your promotional talk will be to introduce yourself as a real-live human being who has a beneficial and a personal service to offer. Your talk should, plainly and succinctly, state what your therapy is, what it might entail, what it could achieve and who may be helped. The substance of your talk, in other words, can be a cut-down version of what may already appear in your publicity brochure but will push the personal angle. Your talk does not need to be a lengthy academic oratory but simply a sincere expression of who you are and what you can offer.

Often the only drawback to giving a promotional talk will be not knowing where to start and, then, as a result, getting a touch of stage-fright. Both of these hurdles can usually be overcome by you especially with practice. For the faint-hearted, it will be advisable for you to keep your talk as short as possible, to provide well-written handouts and to invite questions from your audience. The essence of your talk should be to explain what you do, in simple terms, and you should prepare this aspect well and anticipate questions in this area. Prepare what you are going to say and even rehearse in front of a mirror or before a dummy audience, if necessary.

Often the greatest dread for you may be any on-the-spot questioning. You can, however, avoid this nightmare by inviting your audience-members to consult you privately after your talk, particularly if anyone has any specific questions. By this means, you can buy yourself some thinking-time and you can take yourself momentarily out of the limelight. Be warned, however, that if you do decide to cut the open-forum questioning-session, you could sacrifice an opportunity to answer those questions that many may have but were afraid to ask. Usually your best ploy will be for you to be non-specific in your answer to any question-er that asks specifically about your treatment of a given disease condition or a particular health disorder. In this way, you can shift the focus away from yourself and place the responsibility for healing with your prospective client.

Ask yourself . . .

Can you present yourself as a sincere and caring professional by just being yourself? Can you speak with passion and enthusiasm about your work? Could you carefully plan what you intend to say to your audience? Can you ensure that your talk will be short enough not to bore your audience but long enough to gain their attention and interest? Could you practice your talk in front of a mirror or rehearse with the family listening? Can you anticipate questions and compile a list of stock answers to any questions for your audience? If you are worried about having to answer specific questions, can you find a way of deferring your answers or being non-specific in your replies? Could you provide a case-study example as a means of answering a specific question about your treatment techniques? Could you quote a few well-chosen examples of recovery success as a means of anticipating questions from your audience?

How will you become a competent speaker?

If you need a comforter for the experience of giving a talk, then, take some jottings with you but do not make the mistake of monotonously reading out your notes to your audience. The personal touch, with all its blemishes, will be infinitely more preferably than a stilted and manufactured job.

Discover whether you can gain some inspiration, now, about how to write your notes for a typical promotional presentation. Examine the way in which this task was tackled by a spiritual healer, someone who may well need to quash the general public's many misconceptions about the practice (see Figure 12.1 – *What might a promotional talk on spiritual healing convey?*).

What is spiritual healing?
- a means of addressing health issues naturally
- taps into your body's energy field
- stimulates your own natural healing process
- I become channel for your body's energy to flow
- no ghosts or ghoulies!
- heals mind, body and soul
- supports other healing processes

What does spiritual healing involve?
- you are fully clothed
- you sit in a chair or lie on a coach
- hands-on or slightly above body

What does spiritual healing feel like?
- very relaxing & pleasant
- you may or may not go to sleep
- no limit to number of sessions you can have

Any volunteers?

Any questions?

Hand around brochure & contact details

Figure 12.1 – *What might a promotional talk on spiritual healing convey?*

Another much-misunderstood field might be that of herbal medicine as it may, also, be an area enshrouded in mystery. In the example given below, nothing has been spelled out in full but the practitioner can easily glance down, occasionally, when the flow of his thoughts has been interrupted and he needs a prompt (see Figure 12.2 – *What might a promotional talk on herbal medicine convey?*).

Distribute leaflets and common herbs list

Who am I?
- my background and training
- how I discovered Herbalism

What is herbal medicine?
- strengthens/boosts system and relieves symptoms
- use of the leaves, flowers, stems, berries and roots of plants to prevent, relieve and treat illness
- also known as Phytotherapy
- historic roots from Stone Age, Europe, Far and Middle East
- today's conventional medicines derived from herbal tradition (eg aspirin, codeine, morphine, quinine)
- herbal preps use whole plant and nothing stripped out in laboratory

What does herbal medicine involve?
- extensive case history
- pulse and tongue diagnosis
- iridology – markings on iris and sclera show genetic traits and current state of vital organs
- individual herbs or combinations selected specifically for you – dried, tablets, capsules, lozenges, tinctures, teas, baths, ointments
- wild and farmed herbs
- feed your reactions back to me regularly – monitor progress and adjust preps
- healing crisis

Go through common-herbs list

Invite questions

Figure 12.2 – *What might a promotional talk on herbal medicine convey?*

Always make and keep personal contact with your listeners as much as possible even if you are using notes. Remember that you are selling yourself and, therefore, your personality should shine through in all its glory. Endeavor to be natural and relaxed, regardless of how much of a strange and terrifying ordeal public speaking may be for you. Never be afraid to repeat yourself, possibly, by rephrasing what you have previously stated. In fact, a good ploy might well be to adopt the threefold plan of exposition, development and recapitulation. In other words, you tell them what you intend to tell them, tell them and, then, tell them what you have just told them.

You could embellish your speech with some impressive presentational aids if you have the means of producing some slides cheaply. A number of slides could be used that could act as a prompt for you and might, also, deflect immediate attention away from you if you are feeling nervous about public speaking.

Decide whether you could glean some inspiration from studying a number of slide presentations that have been used by other practitioners in order to accompany a promotional talk. A short slide presentation given by a clinical nutritionist has summed up the topic in a few words (see Figure 12.3 – *What might a slide presentation on clinical nutrition convey?*).

A slide presentation given by a chiropractor has achieved the desired aim as well as adding a human touch to the proceedings (see Figure 12.4 – *What might a slide presentation on McTimoney chiropractic convey?*).

Ask yourself . . .

Can you find a way of writing your speech notes so that you do not risk drying up in mid-flight? Can you write your promotional talk's notes carefully, learn them by heart and, then, discard them on the day? Can you predict what your audience will wish to hear and simultaneously allay any fears or any misconceptions that your participants may have about your practice? Can you anticipate questions by supplying the answers during your speech? Can you inject some humor into your delivery when presenting information to your listeners? Do you have access to a computer with a slide-presentation package so that you could produce some tempting handouts?

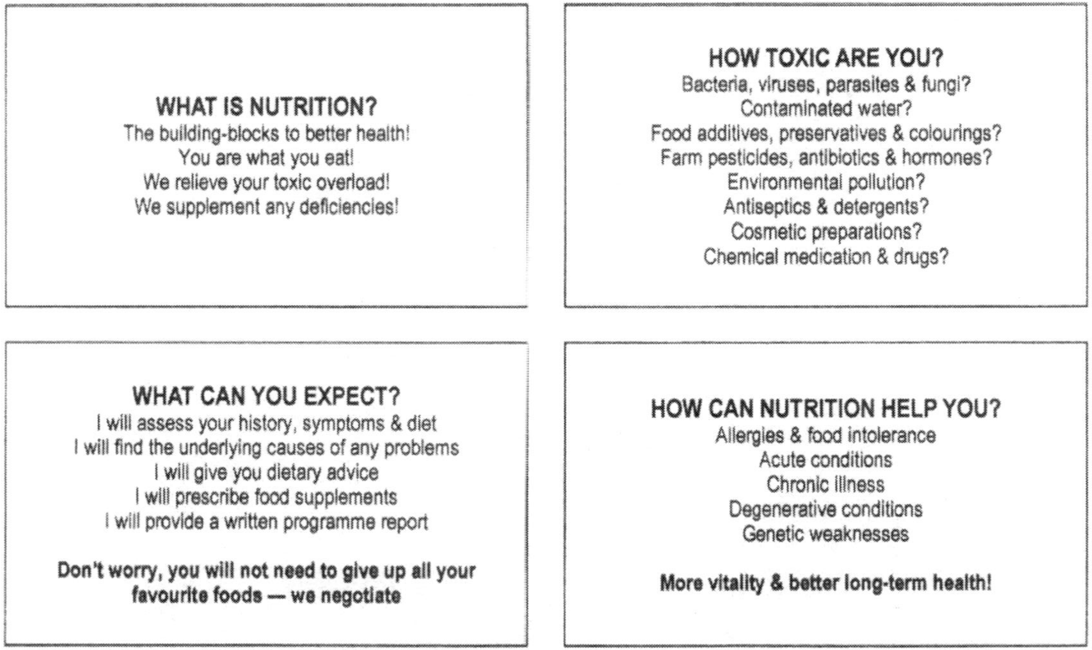

Figure 12.3 – *What might a slide presentation on clinical nutrition convey?*

WHAT IS MCTIMONEY CHIROPRACTIC?
A method of adjusting bones in the body to ensure correct alignment of the spine
Relieves pain and discomfort thus enabling you to live a better quality of life

HOW DOES CHIROPRACTIC WORK?
Speed, dexterity and accuracy of hand movements can accurately make adjustments to realign bones gently but effectively

FACTS ABOUT YOUR SPINE
A misaligned spinal bone could impinge, stretch or compress a spinal nerve resulting in pain, discomfort and restricted mobility
Car accident?
Lifting?
Childbirth?
Poor posture?

HOW CAN CHIROPRACTIC HELP YOU?
McTimoney Chiropractic may improve ...
Back, neck and shoulder pain
Pain, discomfort and stiffness in bones and joints
Migraine and tension headaches
Muscular aches and pains
Sciatica
Whiplash injury
Sports injuries

HOW MANY SESSIONS WILL YOU NEED?
Dependent on ...
The nature of your problem
Your age
How long you have had your problem
Average between 2 and 10 sessions
But remember ...
Prevention is better than cure!

WHAT DO PATIENTS THINK OF CHIROPRACTIC?
McTimoney Chiropractic Association 1997 survey of patients ...
89% "extremely" or "very satisfied" with treatment
85% "very beneficial" for pain management
62% sought treatment for low back pain
93% recommended treatment to family and friends

Figure 12.4 – *What might a slide presentation on McTimoney chiropractic convey?*

How will you follow up your promotional talk?

Whatever you say, and however eloquently you may say it, you may still be advised to give your audience something to take home. If possible, ensure that everyone receives a handout as well as providing all with the opportunity of taking one or two extras for friends. Sometimes those audience-members who were not at all interested in coming to see you personally will, by way of consolation, often become your personal ambassador and will promote your services enthusiastically to others. No-one, therefore, should leave the premises without a handout from you and a winning smile. Your presentation's handout can merely be your brochure, if you have a surfeit of copies, or it can be something tailor-made for the job.

Allow yourself to be inspired by a number of attractive handouts produced by other alternative practitioners. Your handout could purely be a summary of what you have said to your audience designed for your client's future reference as in the case of a talk given by a hypnotherapist (see Figure 12.5 – *What might a handout on hypnotherapy convey?*).

Your handout could, alternatively, be used to give supplementary information to your prospective client that may be too detailed for you to impart during your speech as in the case of a dietary therapist's talk (see Figure 12.6 – *What might a handout on dietary therapy convey?*).

Ask yourself . . .

Will you need any handouts or will your publicity brochure be adequate backup for your promotional talk? Can you be creative with your computer in order to produce some inspirational handout material? Would you need to give out your literature to your audience well in advance of your talk and, then, to draw attention to the contents, at some stage, during your delivery? Can you involve your audience in some practical activity at an appropriate moment? Can you devise a quiz or provide a list of common, treatable ailments that could constitute a memorable handout? Would you be able to give a brief demonstration of what you do in order to show how effective your therapy might be?

Hypnotherapy & Psychotherapy

Would you like to be free of that relentless anguish inside?

What is hypnotherapy?

Hypnotherapy is the utilisation of visualisation and relaxation techniques combined with therapeutic principles. My own therapeutic approach is based on eclectic principles which means that I can draw on a wide range of therapeutic methodology. Therapeutic assistance will allow you to:

- *investigate your past in order to identify the ways in which past traumas and emotional conflicts have impacted on your present*
- *view your current circumstances in context and with insight*
- *understand your unique psychological characteristics and functioning as a whole self-determining personality*
- *modify your irrational thinking-patterns*
- *eliminate your unwanted or unproductive behavioural traits*

How can hypnotherapy help you?

Therapeutic assistance can be of benefit to you in order to naturally alleviate a wide range of distressing symptoms some of which are listed below:

anxiety & panic	*obsessive & compulsive disorders*
bereavement	*post-traumatic stress disorders*
childhood neglect & abuse	*relationship difficulties*
confidence & self-esteem disorders	*sexual dysfunction*
dependencies & addictions	*skin conditions & blushing*
depressive disorders	*sleep disturbances*
eating & digestive disorders	*smoking cessation*
habit & behavioural disorders	*stress & pressure*
irrational fears & phobias	*stuttering & stammering*
migraine & psychosomatic pain	*weight management*

Figure 12.5 – *What might a handout on hypnotherapy convey?*

307

Nutrition and the blood group diet

What's all this about blood groups?

Knowing your blood group can help you to maximize your health, avoid disease, overcome illness, and it can even affect the way you interact with people!

Dr Peter D'Adamo's collection of writing based on extensive scientific research has shown that due to gene linkage each blood group interacts differently with the environment, is susceptible to particular diseases and has distinct emotional needs and preferences. This is hardly surprising if you consider the diverse environments in which they evolved.

O While prehistoric man was hunting and gathering, living mainly on wild game and plants, he developed a very strong muscular body from eating high quality protein. Theories have suggested that group O was the first human blood group.

A Our adept yet spontaneous and unthrifty hunter started running out of animals to eat. Having migrated North from Africa, the hunter had to turn to other means of nourishment for survival. He became more civilized and settled, adapting to his new situation by providing himself with a more dependable diet of cultivated grains and vegetables. As his digestive system evolved to cope so did his blood group, and the co-operative blood group A was born.

B Our ancestor's itchy feet also took him to more remote parts (such as the Himalayas and the Siberian Steppes), where he had to deal with harsh climates and the limitations imposed by traveling. He relied heavily upon his cattle herds for their milk, which he turned into a variety of cultured dairy products. The gene for blood group B started here.

AB The fourth blood group has only existed for about 1000 years, combining the traits of groups A and B when these different cultures started to merge. The modern environment that saw the emergence of group AB lead to the creation of this new blood group through genetic pooling rather than by evolution.

Figure 12.6 – *What might a handout on dietary therapy convey?*

How would you conduct a promotional workshop?

Can you combine self-promotion together with a money-making scheme with your client? One sure-fire way of getting some cash straight into the coffers while, simultaneously, promoting your practice could be to run some group workshops. Certain therapeutic disciplines will lend themselves naturally to this type of activity and, if it would interest you or be appropriate, it could, also, generate much additional business.

Will your therapy offer scope for running a promotional workshop?

Often a series of workshops will generate interest in your practice as well as providing you with some ready cash. During a workshop you will, also, attract your prospective client who may ultimately be seeking a private consultation. Often with a bit of creative thinking, you can dream up a topic or a theme for your workshops that will be self-financing and can go a long way towards promoting your one-to-one sessions. Planning and promoting your workshop should be carefully considered by you both as a marketing tool and as a means of generating finance. Your workshop could be promoted by circulating posters or by compiling a leaflet that specifically advertises this group-activity.

The physically-oriented practices, such as the Alexander technique, Indian head massage, the Pilates method and yoga, can, particularly, lend themselves to the group format. The practitioner of alternative medicine can often use a workshop format in order to explain what would be involved in practices, such as flower essences, herbal medicine, homeopathy and most forms of nutritional therapy. The aim of such a workshop could be to expose your public to what might be on offer and, then, to allow your participants to take away some home-spun remedies. The mind-oriented practices, such as hypnotherapy, life coaching, meditation and neurolinguistic programming, can often provide a small audience with some practical life-survival tools for everyday use. The spiritually-oriented practitioner, similarly, can use a workshop environment in which to banish the popularly-held myths about earth healing, past-life regression, reiki healing, shamanism and most other forms of spiritual healing. Such workshops can frequently bring together like-minded people who may wish to further their spiritual evolution with your assistance.

Ask yourself . . .

Does your therapeutic discipline offer scope for running a workshop? Can you consider running a series of workshops on a given topic closely related to your particular field of practice? Can you design your workshop so that group members can learn about your therapy and, additionally, can undertake some practical work as a sample of what to expect from private treatment? Could you offer to run a series of workshops for a local organization or a neighboring business? Would you be interested in offering an on-going program of workshops? Would you appreciate working in a group setting rather than exclusively offering one-to-one therapy?

What format will your promotional workshop take?

Certain types of therapeutic treatment can be successfully provided in the group setting. In an informal atmosphere, where participants can meet and interact with each other, your prospective client can learn much about your practice and can actually see you in the flesh before taking the plunge and booking a private session. Your workshop should ideally consist of imparting and exchanging information with group-participants as well as providing some practical hands-on activity for all concerned. A workshop could, for instance, be used to impart the philosophy of your practice, to explain the way in which your therapy could be of benefit to your client and, afterwards, to provide an opportunity for your participants to try out your methodology for themselves in an informal setting.

Ask yourself . . .

What kind of information would you endeavor to impart to your workshop-participants? Can you structure your program in such a way that your participants can have ample chance to sample your therapeutic discipline during the workshop sessions? Can you provide your workshop-delegates with some practical work in which they can willingly and constructively engage? Would it be possible for your workshop-participants to take home some free samples or some additional publicity literature? Can you think of an inspiring title for your workshops that will bring in the punters? Can you devise a way of reaching your potential workshop-participants by judicial advertising and promotion? Can you find a suitable venue for your workshops at which you can, also, advertise your services?

How would you practice business networking?

Will you be able to become a dedicated practitioner with your client as well as being a dynamic publicity agent? You may, of course, consider yourself to be a healer rather than a wheeler-dealer but you will, occasionally, need to meet your public. Launching any business may often mean getting yourself noticed and remembered by those people who could prove to be a useful source of contact and referral.

How will you create an atmosphere of fervor?

Develop the habit of talking a lot about what you do with enthusiasm in order to convey the impression that you are a winner at your game. Your mindset will generally create an atmosphere that will draw potential clients to your door.

If you have elected to work in a clinic, then, of course, the first thing you would be advised to do might be to chat up everyone who works there, receptionists and fellow-practitioners alike. If you are working in any form of isolation, then, you will need to do the networking bit in other ways. You could, for instance, join a professional society, such as a business circle or the local chamber of commerce, in which you can meet other business people who may be able to spread the word on your behalf. If your own professional association runs meetings at which you can meet other practitioners in your field, this might provide a valuable source of client-referral for you. You could, perhaps, socialize generally and talk frequently about your work and, then, hand out your brochure, or your business card, to anyone who either may show direct interest or be able to act as your faithful publicity agent.

Another form of networking would be for you to do some foot-slogging. Visit a number of shops and traders in your area and ask if you can display your brochure or if you can leave your business card pinned up on the noticeboard. You could, also, make a round-trip to all the general medical practitioners in your area, and sweet-talk the receptionist, if you do not manage to speak directly to the head honcho. Of course, you will need to call on these people at non-busy times and you must respect the fact that you may need to make an appointment, in advance, or simply wait to be heard. Possibly a mailshot to all local pharmacies and general practitioners would be advisable as an all-purpose publicity tack.

Ask yourself . . .

Can you decide who would be the most appropriate people for you to contact in your area for networking purposes? Would you know intuitively when you might have a nibble at your bait? Can you regard every person you meet as a prospective source of referral? What information can you glean from your local library about likely targets for spreading your word? Are you a good social animal who can talk with enthusiasm about your work? Can you creatively research some hot-spots in your area that may be willing to do some promotional donkey-work on your behalf? Can you drum up some business from your local tennis club or your local ramblers' association?

Would you aspire to a webpage?

Will you need to maintain a robust presence on the internet for your client? The latest publicity stunt will, of course, be to have a webpage about which you can boast to all your friends. Consider, therefore, whether it will be a necessity for you to keep up with your neighbors or whether it would simply be money down the drain.

Will you need a promotional webpage?

Setting up and maintaining your webpage can be a costly luxury that could be prohibitively expensive for you and might not be justified for your practice. The costs of hiring someone to compile, to launch and to maintain your webpage may be right over your humble budget for your small business that caters only for a niche market sector. For this reason, you may well wish to skip to the next section. You may, of course, be able to justify having a webpage, especially if you can design and maintain it yourself without incurring any outlandish expense. If you do not wish to purchase a costly domain name, moreover, you can usually find a tame internet service provider who will donate adequate webspace for virtually nothing.

Before you actually take the plunge and create a website, you may need to seriously consider whether you will get enough business from this form of advertising in order to justify the mega bucks that you may be obliged to spend. If you are working in a large catchment area for prospective punters, and can offer a skill that might be highly in demand, then, you may find that the rewards of a website are well worth the effort and the expense. Consider, furthermore, whether future trends will dictate that not having an internet presence could be fatal for your business.

A halfway house may be for you to add your details to the website of your professional body, your training organization or a site that lists therapeutic services. Often entries on the website of another party can be obtained for little or no cost. If the site is free, then, go for it as you will have nothing to lose. You may find, however, that on the you-pay-for-what-you-get basis, you will not get much for nothing.

Ask yourself . . .

Would a webpage be in keeping with your image? Could you justify the cost of having a webpage for your business? Would a website be an expensive luxury and a financial disaster? Can you afford not to have an internet presence in your area and in your particular profession? Can you manage to get yourself on to someone else's webpage for little or no cost? Can you personally put together a simple webpage for virtually peanuts that does not look cut-price and tacky? Will the future dictate that you should have got there first with your website before the competition catches up with you? If you already have a webpage, can you scour the net for others who might be willing to put a free link to your webpage on their website?

What will your website need to convey?

If you have definitely decided to create your own website and to do it yourself, then, more endless decisions and sleepless nights may be in store for you. Once you have jumped over the maddening hurdle of writing the copy for your brochure, however, cobbling together your website text may be a doddle for you. The wording may not be too much of a headache, if you have already undergone this exercise with your publicity brochure. All you may need to do, now, will be to lift bits out of the text and any pictures from your brochure and, thus, your website can go live. If you are commissioning a specialist in order to design your website, then, you may simply pass your brochure to this third party and, then, go off to lunch.

You will, of course, need to carefully consider the way in which your information will be displayed in a live website-format. Bear in mind that a webpage will have quite a different flavor from the hard copy in your brochure. Maybe you can acquire some inspiration from examining the ways in which other professional practitioners have approached the task of compiling a website. You should, therefore, spend many hours surfing the net and perusing the sites of your colleagues and your competitors in order to decide which approach to take and which tactics to assiduously shun. There may be many jazzy websites out there that blow the mind and influence the senses but few of them would qualify for being appropriate for anyone in a caring profession.

Ask yourself . . .

Can you get a useful friend to design a posh webpage for you for the price of a meal? Could you give a free treatment or two to a kindly webpage designer in return for a favor? Have you carefully considered whether your webpage will portray the right image for you? Can you guarantee that your webpage will be kept up to date? Will your website be the voice with which you will wish to sing to the world? Will your website incorporate an easy way for your prospective client to make contact with you for an initial chat? Will you have a means of monitoring the number of people who might visit your site in order to be able to decipher whether this form of advertising has been cost-effective for your business?

How would you develop your career?

How will you see your own future panning out in front of you after launching your practice? You will not necessarily know where you are going when you initially start up in practice. Often you may be best advised to simply let your practice develop by osmosis. Alternatively, you may wish to give some consideration to your future career and your prospects for professional development.

How will you develop yourself professionally?

As a practising professional, you may well need to supplement your initial training program and, indeed, this may be a requirement of your profession. Many professional associations and regulating bodies in the alternative field will stipulate that practising members must undertake a minimum amount of regular annual training or a degree of self-education in order to meet continuing professional development criteria. Over and above this minimal stipulation, you may, also, wish to consider what your personal training needs might be for your own advancement.

Further training will often constitute self-development for you and, therefore, you should welcome the opportunity rather than regarding it as a necessary evil. You should, of course, give careful consideration to which training activities you will elect to undertake. Sometimes, as a newly-qualified practitioner, you will become obsessed with taking additional training courses and the habit can be both exhausting as well as being very expensive. Do not, however, be tempted to retake your initial training course in the hope that you will get it right the second time around. Your working experience will usually be sufficient to allay most of your unwarranted fears. You should only undertake an additional training course in areas of special interest for you in order to explore ways of self-development and practice development. Signing up for every training course that has been advertised could become a full-time money-wasting and time-wasting exercise.

Often a practitioner in one field will decide to expand into a closely-related area of expertise because some disciplines will naturally go hand in hand. Your practice methodology will inevitably alter many times along your career path. The way in which you will work and you might deal with your client today will, without doubt, be vastly different from what it might have been when you first started out in practice. Your training requirements, now, moreover, will look utterly different in years to come. Observe your own progress and, thus, learn from your experience in practice.

Ask yourself . . .

Do you see yourself needing any further training over and above any statutory profession-specific requirements? Do you intend to specialize in a given aspect of your work and, so, you should enhance your skills in that specific area? Do you need to undertake an advanced course in order to ensure expertise in your particular field? What might be your general reaction to compulsory continuing professional development? Do you feel that there could be any gap in your knowledge that you would wish forthwith to plug? Do you have a special skill that you would like to perfect? What aspects of your work might interest you the most as a healing professional? Have you decided to study for a sister-qualification that is closely related to your existing skill? Have you considered in which direction your career will ultimately develop? Are you quite content to jog along happily doing what you are doing both, now, and for the foreseeable future? What have you learned about professional practice from your past experience? What does your professional body have to offer in terms of cost-effective additional training? Would a specialist training course in an up-and-coming topic be an advantage to your business?

Let's take an example – Gertrude's story

Gertrude became insatiably interested in exploring the whole field of alternative healing but not with any particular intention of becoming a practitioner. Gertrude, thus, found herself taking a number of short taster-courses merely out of interest. Gertrude explored reflexology, the metamorphic technique, Indian head massage, thermo-auricular therapy, Bach flower remedies, reiki healing and crystal healing. While testing the water in this way, Gertrude realized that her natural curiosity had made her something of an expert in the field. Because of this burgeoning proficiency, Gertrude was soon asked to teach reflexology at her local adult education center and it was, then, that she received her wakeup call.

Gertrude saw this turn of events as a positive sign that she should, now, become fully qualified in her chosen field, principally in reflexology and healing, and, by this time, she felt able to determine her own future and to see her path ahead clearly. Once Gertrude had become qualified as a practitioner, she, then, found her training and education was further enhanced by the obligation to undertake continuing professional development courses. Gertrude's horizons, thus, expanded still further while she watched her career continually evolving and ultimately she became a trail-blazer in developing an entirely new healing technique as an off-shoot of reflexology.

Let's take an example – Mercutio's story

Mercutio trained as an acupuncturist and started his therapeutic practice soon after qualifying. To his amazement, Mercutio found that his very first client was at death's door and that there was virtually nothing he could do in order to save her. Mercutio discovered that his client wished earnestly to die in her own home, despite the fact that her family were urging her to go into a hospice. This dilemma stirred up much soul-searching for Mercutio who did not yet have the experience to deal with this unusual situation.

Inevitably, Mercutio's client passed away and naturally Mercutio felt a keen sense of personal failure as well as harboring a feeling of apprehension about what her relatives might think of his treatment strategies. As it turned out, however, the relatives of Mercutio's deceased client were full of praise for his part in the proceedings and commended him highly for allowing her to die in the place of her choice. Mercutio, thus, realized that his own perception of events could be at complete variance with those of others. Moreover, Mercutio appreciated that his personal efforts could, in no way, magically determine the outcome of his client's treatment to his satisfaction.

The important lessons that Mercutio learned were invaluable to him especially, now, that he has become a teacher of acupuncture who passes his wisdom on to his pupils. Mercutio, latterly, stresses to his trainees that personal perception is simply that – just personal – and that all the practitioner can ever do will be to merely await the outcome over which he will have no absolute control. Here, then, is an example of the way in which a practitioner can learn by being thrown in at the deep end but can, subsequently, pass such wisdom on to others in a beneficial way.

Where would your career be going in the future?

What do you imagine the future will really hold for you and your business? Get to know yourself well enough in order to decide what kind of business animal you actually could be as an individual. This introduction to yourself will stand you in good stead when focusing on your business and when enhancing your personal future.

How will you further your career path?

As far as business expansion might be concerned, you may need to give some thought to the ways in which you could broaden your horizons in the long term. You may be content with your lot for many years to come and, if so, fine. If you know yourself to be one who will search for greener pastures, then, maybe, meditate on where you are going in the future. Decide whether you are the entrepreneurial type who will want to open your own multi-disciplinary practice and, then, employ others to work for you. Choose whether you will want to move to offices in a more prestigious area where all the posh people hang out.

In addition to conducting your therapeutic work, you may, also, wish to consider other ways of raking in the cash while, simultaneously, promoting your business. Decide whether you will want to teach, to supervise or to write books. Becoming a supervisor in your chosen profession can further your ability to help others as well as adding much interest to your life's work. Think about whether you will want to sell some of your ideas or your inventions in order to assist other practitioners. In certain professions, you may be able to sell products, such as supplements, remedies, tapes or other self-help aids, to your client.

Often a modicum of creative thinking and entrepreneurial flare can inspire you to develop your business effectively. You may find that you can capitalize on previous experience in order to be able to offer a unique service to other practitioners. Obvious examples of any marketable skills in the alternative profession might be bookkeeping services, marketing advice, secretarial services, the supply of therapeutic aids and webpage design.

Ask yourself . . .

How do you envisage the expansion of your business over the next 5 to 10 years? Do you consider that you will have the desire to expand your horizons once you have got your practice well and truly up and running? Will you get itchy feet in a couple of years and will you need to broaden your perspective? Do you have aspirations to teach, to run a therapy center or to invent a new product? Could you invest in premises and, then, hire this accommodation out to other practitioners? Might there be any way in which you could put a new slant on what you do in order to steal a march on the competition? Can you see yourself in a novel way of working and, then, share this knowledge with others? Do you have a marketable skill that you could sell to other practitioners? Would you enjoy and have a natural ability to supervise other practitioners in your field? How will you move yourself forward along your personal evolutionary path? In what ways have you personally benefited from the wisdom contained within this book? Can you wish yourself every happiness for the future?

ABOUT THE AUTHOR

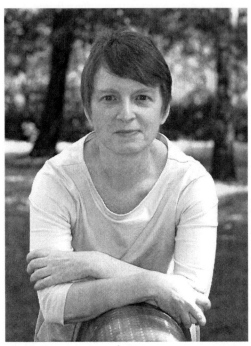

Jacquelyne Morison is an analytical hypnotherapist, a craniosacral therapist, a nutritional therapist and an energetic healer. Jacquelyne has been in private practice since 1995 and, formerly, she worked in Harley Street in London.

Jacquelyne is a visiting trainer at the **Institute of Clinical Hypnotherapy & Psychotherapy** (Republic of Ireland) and the **International College of Eclectic Therapies** (London).

Jacquelyne is a supervisor of practising therapists in various disciplines and is an accredited Supervisory Skills Training Provider for the National Council for Psychotherapists in the UK.

Jacquelyne is, also, the author of the highly acclaimed work **Analytical Hypnotherapy Volume 1: Theoretical Principles** (2001, ISBN 1899836772) and **Volume 2: Practical Applications** (2002, ISBN 1899836853) both published by Crown House Publishing Limited.

Printed in the United Kingdom by
Lightning Source UK Ltd., Milton Keynes
136903UK00002B/56/P